WOMEN'S EXPERIENCE OF BREAST FEEDING

Heather Maclean

WOMEN'S EXPERIENCE OF B·R·E·A·S·T F·E·E·D·I·N·G

UNIVERSITY OF TORONTO PRESS
Toronto Buffalo London

© University of Toronto Press 1990
Toronto Buffalo London
Printed in Canada

ISBN 0-8020-6756-5

Printed on acid-free paper

Canadian Cataloguing in Publication Data

Maclean, Heather, 1947–
Women's experience of breast feeding

Includes bibliographical references.
ISBN 0-8020-6756-5

1. Breast feeding – Ontario – Toronto. I. Title.

RJ216.M33 1990   649'.3'09713541   c89-095064-4

Dedicated to David, my son,
with whom I shared the
pleasure of breast feeding

Contents

PREFACE ix
ACKNOWLEDGMENTS xi

Part One   Introduction
1 The Social Influences on Breast Feeding 3
2 Study Rationale and Methods 8

Part Two   Making Feeding Choices
3 Choosing to Breast Feed 19
4 Choosing to Bottle Feed 25

Part Three   The Realities of Breast Feeding
5 The Physical Discomforts 35
6 Assessing the Milk Supply 45

7 Feeding Schedules 57
8 Fatigue 69
9 Time Commitments 72
10 Breast Feeding in Public 83
11 The Rewards of Breast Feeding 95

Part Four Weaning

12 The Decision to Wean Early 113
13 Reasons for Early Weaning 123
14 Weaning between Four Months and One Year 136

Part Five Support Networks

15 Breast Feeding in the Hospital 147
16 Physicians 157
17 Family Relationships 172
18 Other Sources of Support 194

Part Six Conclusion

19 Promoting Breast Feeding 203

REFERENCES 213
INDEX 219

Preface

This book is written both for professionals who work with women who intend to or are breast feeding and for women who are pregnant or in the midst of nursing. It documents the findings of a major, prospective study of women's experience of breast feeding and presents a detailed and integrated picture of breast feeding, using the words of the women themselves to convey the nature and meaning of this important event.

The book offers a window on breast feeding for professionals, particularly those who have not experienced either breast feeding or motherhood. It should help them to develop a better understanding of the range of factors influencing the quality of breast feeding and the range of strategies that are needed to promote it. The book will also be of interest to women who are considering breast feeding. It is hoped that the content will prepare women for what may unfold and encourage them, and society as a whole, to recognize the work of mothering. Taking care of a baby (of which breast feeding is a central feature) is a craft that deserves acknowledgment and support. Women who are breast feeding will find the book a handy reference. They will learn they are not alone in their feelings; others have walked the path before them and this is their legacy.

In some respects, this book is as much about what it is like to have a baby as it is about breast feeding. Many of the challenges described by our study participants would be shared by women who bottle feed. None the less, breast feeding does contribute a special dimension to mothering. It places added time demands on the mother. It changes her body. It ties her to her infant. It generates strong reactions from others. But most of all, it offers a mysterious and unique opportunity for a special way to nurture. As women, we are privileged to be able to breast feed. We must therefore ensure that all of us do what we can to foster an environment that enables women and babies to share the rewards of breast feeding.

The issues presented in the book reflect a wide spectrum of data. Some were of concern to almost everyone; others were of concern to a few; together they provide a comprehensive framework. Because this was a qualitative study we were not specifically concerned with quantifying responses or patterns. Nevertheless, an attempt is made to indicate whether given concerns were common or rare within the group interviewed. As well, throughout the text words are used that imply magnitude, such as majority, many, most, some, and a few. In general, these terms are defined as follows: few – recurrent but reported by less than 10–15 per cent of the interviewees; some – more than a few but less than 25–30 per cent; many – a substantial minority but less than a majority; most – more than a majority. These terms sometimes refer to the entire group of 100 women. At other times they refer to a specific category as indicated by the context. These words represent our best judgment of frequency but may not necessarily reflect an actual count.

The quotations used throughout have sometimes been abridged or slightly altered to fit the flow. Always, the spirit of the speaker is retained. Pseudonyms have been used to protect the confidentiality of the people we interviewed.

Acknowledgments

This book is the culmination of a large study of women's experience of breast feeding that took place in Toronto, Canada, over a four-year period. The study would not have been possible without the commitment of the 122 women who were interviewed, especially the 50 women who participated in up to fourteen interviews each. I am grateful for their generosity in giving their time and viewpoints during that hectic period before and after the baby's birth. The interviewing process can be intense and demanding for both the interviewee and the interviewer. I would like to express my appreciation to Rosemary Gray-Snelgrove, Sue Ferrier, Marianne Williams, Barbara Oram, Lynne Kirkwood, Christine Marshall, and Mickey Wischnewski for the energy and commitment they devoted to the interviewing.

I am indebted to many people who contributed to the administrative and analytic facets of the study. Rosemary Gray-Snelgrove was project co-ordinator for three years and Sue Ferrier, who was with the project almost from start to finish, was project co-ordinator for the last year. Elizabeth Fry, Naseem Janmohamed, and Linda Pickard assisted with the analysis. Stefa Katamay, along with Sue Ferrier, helped draft portions of the project report that served as the blueprint for this book. Mary Ferguson was a study participant and research assistant and gently but repeatedly encouraged me to write this book.

This project has required an enormous amount of secretarial support and I would like to acknowledge the work of Irene Staggopoulos, Laurie Short, and Linda Hoogakker and the Word Processing Centre of the Faculty of Medicine, University of Toronto. I am also grateful for the support of my co-investigator Niall Byrne, and for the thoughtful and constructive critical assistance of my colleague George Beaton. I would like to acknowledge as well the physicians and nurses at Women's College Hospital, Mount Sinai Hospital, and the Toronto General Hospital for their assistance with recruitment.

This research was supported by a National Health Research and Development Program Grant no. 6606-1940-46. I am indebted to the program not only for the financial support but also for its generous encouragement of a new researcher.

An earlier version of chapter 19 originally appeared in *Health Promotion* 3 (1989): 361–70.

Finally, I wish to thank my son David Bates and my husband Don Maudsley, each of whom, in his own way, has helped me keep perspective on projects that never seem to end.

Heather Maclean
Toronto, June 1989

PART ONE

Introduction

CHAPTER ONE

The Social Influences on Breast Feeding

This book reports the findings of an extensive study of women's experience of breast feeding. The purpose of the study was to examine breast feeding from the perspective of those who know it best: women themselves.

Breast feeding, as one woman who was interviewed said, 'is the epitome of motherhood.' It is surrounded by an aura of romance and sentimentality. It is natural and instinctive. It creates feelings that cannot be matched by other forms of interaction. It is the ultimate gift. Every woman should choose to breast feed. In some respects these statements are true. Breast feeding can be a truly wonderful experience. There are many compelling reasons why it is a good thing to do. Why, then, are there problems with breast feeding? Why do so many women give up before they have barely begun? The answers to these questions lie in understanding the context in which breast feeding occurs. Women's beliefs, attitudes, and experiences do not develop in isolation. They reflect not only a woman's unique personality and preferences but also the social forces and viewpoints that are a part of the world in which she lives. Throughout the last century, women's attitudes on the merits of breast and bottle feeding have reflected changing viewpoints in society. The trend to bottle feeding developed at a time when science and technology were viewed as solutions to the world's problems. Science could improve on nature, and mothers around the world – wanting to do what was best for their children – switched to infant formula. By the middle 1950s, a whole set of social norms, centred on technology and the knowledge of experts, developed around the management of pregnancy, delivery, and child raising. By the late 1960s and early 1970s, a grass-roots scepticism of science and technology had developed, especially among the well-educated but disillusioned youth of industrialized countries. Women began to question the utility and effectiveness of high-technology medical interventions to control their reproductive systems and there was a growing concern about the medicalization of childbirth. A rekindled interest in breast feeding was a natural outgrowth of this shifting socio-cultural milieu. The tide had turned and mothers who wanted to do the best for their children embraced breast feeding. This shift, however, has not been achieved without difficulty. It has taken place in an environment that still, in large measure, adheres to the values of the previous era. Large numbers of women who have moved into the flow have been caught in the rip-tide.

The purpose of this book is to ground our knowledge of breast feeding in women's realities. Women's experience is an overlooked source of wisdom about the nature of our lives. It is a wisdom that needs to be shared among us. This shared information is *not* intended to discourage women from breast feeding. It is meant to prepare them for what is to come and to demonstrate that difficulties and challenges are an inherent and legitimate part of mothering. The difficulties women experience when breast feeding are not problems they have brought upon themselves because they are inadequate to the task but are consequences of the work of mothering and also of the social norms of our culture.

Many women are disillusioned when their experience of breast feeding does not measure up to their idealized expectations. The romantic images are frequently divorced from the everyday reality of caring for a baby in much the same way that the romantic image of love excludes the struggles and efforts that are necessary to nurture it. It is assumed that women will lovingly embrace all the tasks entailed in mothering an infant, when, in fact, all too often women are ill prepared for the reality of that experience. Many women are dismayed to discover how much work goes into caring for a baby and breast feeding. This response is not surprising because the nature of mothers' work has rarely been documented. Given our current tendency to equate work with remuneration, mothering is sometimes not considered 'work' at all.

Much of the professional literature on breast feeding has stressed education as a strategy to help women breast feed for longer periods of time. Without denying the importance of education, this emphasis may be misplaced. Breast feeding takes place in a social milieu that promotes and idealizes breast feeding. This same milieu encourages women to believe that everything in life is within their individual control. It idolizes the superwoman; it glamorizes paid work and undervalues domestic work; it glorifies women's breasts as sex objects but abhors public displays of breast feeding; it reveres thin bodies over maternal shapes; and it relegates the responsibilities of child bearing and rearing to the private realm of the family. To understand the factors that influence women's experience of breast feeding it is necessary to understand the influence of these socio-cultural factors that reflect women's place in society. If we want to encourage more women to breast feed and to enhance the quality of the experience of those who do, we must press for social change as well as individual change. The promotion of breast feeding requires political efforts to change the social milieu so it is more supportive of women's needs. In the meantime, women who experience problems breast feeding must understand that they are not alone in their difficulties, nor are they at fault. Difficulties are inevitable. The post-partum period is characterized by remarkable changes: changes in attitudes, feelings, and values, in physical and emotional energy, in appearance, in relationships, and in roles.

This book documents the character of breast feeding. It traces the range of experiences and reactions that women have over the course of breast feeding. It illustrates how social forces interact with personal factors to shape the nature of the experience. It presents the trials and tribulations, the wonder and the joys, using the thoughts and words of women who were in the midst of the experience.

The participants in our study spoke about every facet of breast feeding. They discussed at length the day-to-day realities of breast feeding: the baby's temperament, the baby's feeding schedule, the impact of the frequent feedings, the daily difficulties of coping, the discomfort of breast feeding in the early stages, and the overwhelming fatigue. They described their feelings about breast feeding: their reaction to carrying the sole responsibility for feeding, their feelings about being tied down, their concerns about the changes in their bodies and their lives, and the pleasures derived from this special form of nurturing. They also discussed the choices they faced as they coped with the ups and downs of breast feeding. Should they feed by schedule or on demand? Did they have sufficient milk? Should they add a formula supplement? Should they introduce a bottle to ensure they could have some time away from the baby? Where could they breast feed away from home with relative ease? When the feeding is going badly should they wean? When has a baby been breast fed long enough? Finally, women described their interaction with others: their partners, members of their immediate families and other relatives, friends, neighbours, and health professionals. Women spoke of how these people helped or hindered breast feeding and the degree of support they offered. These topics are all discussed in detail in this book.

The book is divided into five parts. The study methods are described in the second chapter of part one. Part two describes how women made the decision to breast or bottle feed and examines the factors that influenced that decision. Part three presents the character of breast feeding, including what it entails and women's reactions to it. It documents the physical discomfort, approaches to feeding, fatigue, the time constraints, concerns about the milk supply, and women's views and experiences of breast feeding in public. Part four addresses weaning. It describes the events that led to early weaning and the reactions women had to stopping prematurely. It also describes the experience of weaning between four months and one year of age, including why and how women weaned and their reactions to it. Part five looks at the role of others and their support (or lack of) for the breast-feeding mother. In part six, the concluding chapter summarizes the book by looking at how a new baby changes the mother's world and examines what can be done to enhance the quality of breast feeding for all women.

CHAPTER TWO

Study Rationale and Methods

Since the late 1970s the professional literature on breast feeding has mushroomed. There have been a host of studies, conducted within a broad spectrum of disciplines, on physiological, psychological, and socio-cultural aspects of breast feeding. There has been a particular interest in documenting feeding practices, and in examining the determinants of decisions to breast or bottle feed and to stop breast feeding prematurely.

Recent History of Breast Feeding

Prior to 1920, 90 per cent of Canadian mothers breast fed their babies (Yeung, Pennell, Leung, and Hall 1981). After that time the number of women breast feeding dropped dramatically so that by 1963 it was estimated that only 30–40 per cent of women initiated breast feeding. This figure changed little over the next ten years (Health and Welfare Canada 1982; Myres 1979; McNally, Hendricks, and Horowitz 1985). Jelliffe (1976) and Jelliffe and Jelliffe (1978, 1981) have written extensively about possible reasons for this decline. These include:
- rapid urbanization and industrialization accompanied by an attitude that technological developments are superior to natural processes

- the changing role of women in society with a concomitant increase in the number of women working outside the home
- adoption of the cultural attitude in which women's breasts are valued exclusively for aesthetic and erotic reasons, not for their nurturing function
- marketing advertising, and promotion of infant formula
- insufficient action by government to promote breast feeding
- insufficient emphasis and understanding of breast feeding by health professionals

By 1973, however, a major shift in breast-feeding rates was beginning. The shift occurred in two waves that peaked between 1973 and 1978 and between 1981 and 1982. Surveys by Ross Laboratories indicated that national breast-feeding rates increased during these waves by 69 per cent and 15 per cent respectively (McNally et al. 1985). This shift has been attributed to changed attitudes in industrialized societies protesting the over-mechanization of modern life-styles, renewed interest in conservation and ecology, critical scrutiny of the infant-formula industry, developments in scientific knowledge related to breast milk, and increased advocacy by health professionals (Jelliffe and Jelliffe 1978, 1981).

From 1982 until 1987 (the last year for which figures are available) the rates have shifted up and down by three or four percentage points (Ross Laboratories, personal communication, 31 January 1989). In 1987, 80 per cent of the women sampled elected to breast feed. These rates were national averages and therefore varied by region. Rates in Quebec and Atlantic Canada trailed significantly behind those of the other provinces. In Quebec the 1987 in-hospital breast-feeding rate was 66 per cent (up from 60 per cent in 1983) and in Atlantic Canada the rate was 72 per cent (up from 57 per cent in 1983).

The Ross Laboratories surveys also show that Canadian women are continuing to breast feed for longer periods of time, a trend that is confirmed by studies by McNally et al. (1985) and Tanaka, Yeung, and Anderson (1987). The number of mothers stopping breast feeding within the critical first two months is now half of what it was in 1973. None the less, there is still cause for concern. The 1987 figures indicate that, of the sample of women who started breast feeding, 17.5 per cent had stopped by two months, 41 per cent had stopped by four months, and 60 per cent had stopped by six months (Ross Laboratories, personal communication, 31 January 1989). Although the cessation rates have decreased, they are still high when compared to the Canadian Paediatric Society (1978, 1979) recommendation that breast milk should be the only source of nutrients for most infants for the first three to six months of life. The Ross survey showed that in 1987 only 66, 47, and 32 per cent of babies at two, four, and six months of age respectively were being breast fed (Ross Laboratories, personal communication, 31 January 1989). Clearly, if we wish to encourage women to breast feed for longer periods of time, we must develop a better understanding of the factors that influence women's experience of this process.

Factors Affecting Choice and Duration of Breast Feeding

Simopolous and Grave (1984) in a comprehensive review of the factors influencing the choice and duration of breast feeding noted that the reasons for early termination are vague and poorly understood. It is acknowledged that physical, psychological, and social factors are all important but 'the issue is complex, involving extensive social, economic, and motivational factors' (Simopoulos and Grave 1984: 603). The authors highlighted the importance of a number of factors, including the level of the parents' education, family income and socio-economic status, parity, employment status of the mother, presence or absence of social networks, social taboos on breast feeding in public, mother's attitudes and values, mother's health status, and hospital practices.

Research Approaches

Most research on breast-feeding practices takes the form of

surveys where questionnaires are either mailed or administered in person to the mother on a one-time-only basis. There are important limitations to survey research, particularly in the way in which it over-simplifies complex processes. The structured format of questionnaires channels respondents' thinking along certain lines and discourages them from conceptualizing and elaborating for themselves the factors they perceive to be important (Maclean 1989a). Responses to questionnaires can fail to illuminate the underlying reasons for certain attitudes and behaviour that are central to a thorough understanding of breast feeding (Quandt 1985; Sjolin, Hofvander, and Hillervik 1977, 1979; Van Esterik and Greiner 1981).

A number of researchers have noted the need for more studies that follow women over the course of breast feeding (Allen and Pelto 1985; Chapman, Macey, Keegan, Borum, and Bennett 1985; Graef, McGhee, Rozycki, Fescina-Jones, Clark, Thompson, and Brooten 1988; Simopoulos and Grave 1984; Sjolin et al. 1977; Tully and Dewey 1985). Breast feeding occurs many times a day, every day, over a period of months. To understand it thoroughly it must be examined in a way that captures its changing patterns.

Other researchers support such an approach and, in addition, call for the use of qualitative methods that allow women to identify and articulate the nature of their own experience (Adair 1983; Hewat and Ellis 1984; Lee and Solimano 1981; Sjolin et al. 1979). This approach allows the researcher to study breast feeding within its larger context. Breast feeding does not take place in isolation. It is an integral part of the experience of having a new baby and its meaning is dependent on the mother's experience of pregnancy, birth, and the postnatal period.

One of the significant gaps in the professional literature on breast feeding is the absence of a comprehensive picture of the range of factors that influence breast feeding, especially one that integrates the personal influences with socio-cultural ones. Because social forces are expressed in personal decisions and actions of members of a culture or society, the interaction between the two must be studied together.

The study described in this book was developed to redress some of the gaps in our understanding of breast feeding and to suggest strategies that might enable women to breast feed for longer periods of time. The specific methods used in this study and a description of the sample are described below.

Study Methods

The objectives of this study on women's experience of breast feeding were threefold: to examine the factors that influence women's decision to breast or bottle feed; to understand the factors that lead women to stop breast feeding early (within four months of delivery) and, conversely, to identify the factors that encourage women to continue breast feeding for longer periods; and, finally, to examine the degree and nature of support women experience within the family and the broader community. The fundamental premise underlying the three objectives was the importance of examining these factors through a thorough understanding of the perspectives and experiences of women who were breast feeding.

The method employed in this study is called interpretive phenomenology. This method has much in common with other qualitative methods in the social sciences, such as ethnography, ethnomethodology, and symbolic interactionism; all emphasize understanding the point of view of the person being studied. They are concerned with comprehending the meanings of actions and events from the participant's frame of reference as a means of illuminating the interaction of personal and contextual factors that shape behaviour. A number of sources served as the methodological basis of the study (Bogdan and Taylor 1975; Bogdan and Biklen 1982; Giorgi 1970; Glaser and Strauss 1967; Keen 1975; Sullivan 1984).

The study sample consisted of 100 pregnant volunteers who intended to breast feed and 22 women who either intended to or were bottle feeding. The women were recruited into the study through brochures placed in obstetricians' offices, family-practice units, and pre-natal clinics that were associated with three downtown Toronto teaching hospitals affiliated with the Faculty of Medicine, University of Toronto. Half the women intending to breast feed were randomly assigned to the study group. They were interviewed once in the third trimester of pregnancy and then twelve times between the birth of their baby and six months post-partum. Women who were still breast feeding at one year were interviewed again at that time. Seven interviews were conducted in person and seven by telephone. If a woman stopped breast feeding prior to six months the interviews were terminated. The remaining fifty women who were intending to breast feed were interviewed twice in person, once in the third trimester and once at six months post-partum. An interview guide was used to conduct the first and last interviews with women in both groups. The remaining interviews with the fifty women in the study group were less structured; the intention was to encourage them to describe and discuss their experience of breast feeding. The women who were intending to bottle feed or who were bottle feeding were interviewed in the third trimester or within five weeks of the baby's birth. An interview guide was used to focus the interviews.

All the interviews were tape-recorded and transcribed. In total there were 756 interviews and over 20,000 pages of transcripts. Via methods common to qualitative analysis, the transcripts were coded according to categories and themes (Bogdan and Biklen 1982; Giorgi 1970; Glaser and Strauss 1967; Patton 1980; Spradley 1979; Taylor and Bogdan 1984). A computer program was developed to assist with category sorting, which preceded a detailed interpretive analysis of the data.

Study Participants

The breast-feeding participants in this study were similar to the larger population of Canadian women who breast feed their babies. In comparison with the general population of women who give birth, women who breast feed tend to be better educated and have relatively high family incomes (Health and Welfare Canada 1982; Myres 1979; McNally et al. 1985; Yeung et al. 1981). Of the breast-feeding women in this study, 85 per cent had completed all or some post-secondary education; 66 per cent had annual combined family incomes greater than the average Canadian family income; 76 per cent were aged 26–35 years; 97 per cent were married or living in partnership with the father; and 51 per cent had at least one other child (and all but one had prior breast-feeding experience). Sixty per cent of the participants were born in Canada and 67 per cent of the group had lived in Canada for ten years or longer. The sample of bottle-feeding women was less well educated (only 38 per cent had some post-secondary education), had lower combined family incomes (only 47 per cent had incomes greater than the Canadian average), and a larger percentage had more than one child (73 per cent).

As will be seen later in this book, the women in this study breast fed for a much longer time period than the majority of Canadian women. This would suggest that the women who volunteered for the study were somehow different from the average Canadian who breast feeds (despite the surface similarities) or that ongoing participation in the study encouraged women to breast feed longer. The study was designed in such a way that the latter possibility could be examined. Half the women were interviewed regularly over a six-month period but the other half were interviewed only twice. The duration of breast feeding was almost identical in both groups, indicating that repeated interviewing was not a factor in the prolonged breast feeding. It is more likely that volunteers who participate in this type of research project may be more highly motivated and more committed to breast feeding than those who do not volunteer.

Despite the fact that these women breast fed considerably longer than average, their experience sheds a good deal of light on the subject of breast feeding. A great many of them encountered difficulties that might overwhelm women with less determination. As well, because of their higher levels of education and income, they may have had more access to information sources and other forms of support. The pictures presented by these women are likely 'best-case' scenarios, which underscore the need for ongoing action to ensure that all women will have the opportunity to breast feed successfully.

PART TWO

Making Feeding Choices

The number of women choosing to breast feed has increased dramatically in the last fifteen to twenty years. The participants in this study demonstrated the degree to which many women are now aware of and believe in the benefits of breast feeding. Indeed, for half our sample, breast feeding had become so much a part of the maternity culture that the choice was made without thought. Breast feeding was simply what one did. The other half of the women made their decision after giving considerable thought to the advantages and disadvantages of breast feeding. They learned about the advantages to the baby's health and the convenience. They were drawn to it because it was natural and because it provided an opportunity for enhanced closeness between mother and child.

It was more difficult to investigate the reasons for bottle feeding. Despite extensive efforts, we could not find many women intending to bottle feed who were willing to talk with us. We think this reluctance may have resulted partly from the fact that these women believed they were doing something that contravened current social norms. Those we spoke with did not take the decision to bottle feed lightly. They knew about the benefits of breast feeding but concluded that, on balance, it was better for them to bottle feed. Many of these women expressed concern about displaying their breasts in public. They were eager to see their bodies return to normal and were reluctant to be tied too heavily to the demands of their infants. They were aware that they were moving against the tide of popular opinion but believed that meeting their own needs was not going to compromise seriously the well-being of their babies. In many cases, their own previous experience has affirmed that belief.

CHAPTER THREE

Choosing to Breast Feed

Why Women Breast Fed

All the women we spoke to were very aware of the benefits of breast feeding. Their reasons for breast feeding were similar to those identified in other studies (Adair 1983; Fieldhouse 1982; Florak, Oberman-DeBoer, Van Kampen-Donker, Van Wingen, and Kromhout 1984; Yeung et al. 1981). The women we interviewed discussed its nutritional advantages, the health benefits of the antibodies, enhanced oral development associated with sucking, bacteriological safety, the naturalness of mother's milk, the shrinking effect on the uterus, the ease and convenience of feeding, the intimacy, and the satisfaction of providing 'the best' for the baby. The following comment is typical: 'It seems obvious to me that breast milk is what the baby should have. Why bother spending a lot of money on formula if you've got a supply there anyhow. There's also the matter of antibodies. And it always seemed to me an enormous amount of trouble and bother to sterilize bottles. I guess also that it creates a closeness between mother and baby that I just don't think you can get any other way.'

A striking feature of the comments was the strength of the conviction that breast feeding was, quite simply, 'the best.'

There was no doubt in the minds of these women that breast milk was 'better than' formula. Over and over women reiterated this viewpoint: 'I believe that it's obviously better for the baby.' / 'The mother's milk is a lot better and has a lot more preventive medicine in it for the baby.' / 'I don't want to give my child formula because breast milk is so much healthier.'

Of all the reasons given for breast feeding the most common were its naturalness, the ease and convenience, the intimacy, and personal satisfaction. *Webster's Ninth New Collegiate Dictionary* defines 'natural' as based on an inherent sense of right and wrong and as being in accordance with nature. Both these definitions capture the significance that breast feeding held for many women: 'It just seemed like the most natural thing to do.' / 'Breast feeding is the most natural, the most obvious and the best gift, really, that we can give a baby.' / 'Nature always knows best. Breast feeding a baby is probably the epitome of womanhood.'

Women assumed that breast feeding was easy and convenient. For some this perception was based on previous experience: 'I chose to breast feed for the reason of convenience. I can't imagine having to prepare formula and get bottles sterilized and have it all stocked up in the fridge and go through that sort of thing.' Many women who were expecting their first child also anticipated that breast feeding would be convenient. As one mother said: 'It looks like it's more of a pain to bottle feed.' As we will see later, a few of these women found post-birth that breast feeding was not always as convenient or as easy as they had anticipated, particularly if they encountered major difficulties.

The most common reason for breast feeding was the belief that it enhanced the degree of intimacy between the baby and the mother.

I think breast feeding is a means of nurturing the child. Not only does a baby need food but he needs the warmth and the security. Holding a baby in your arms and feeding him at the same time supplies a lot of the needs he has.

I have already breast fed. I was successful at it and liked the closeness. I thought that it was very important and it's not something I'd like to give up on unless I really had to.

I think the main reason for me is psychological — that closeness and wanting to really cuddle a baby and, I suppose, the giving of yourself.

Many women used the word 'bonding' to describe the developing intimacy and believed that it was promoted by breast feeding: 'You develop a bond with your child by breast feeding. I get almost weepy when I see mothers and their babies. It's such a touching thing, very emotional.' / 'As you look after your child — that's how bonding develops. You're really close to your baby when you're breast feeding. You feel like you're giving yourself to the baby — what else do you want, what else could you do?'

There was the sense that breast feeding represented a gift, a giving of oneself for the betterment of another: 'You are satisfied. Breast feeding feels good. You know you are doing your best, you just do anything you can to make the baby happy.' As this gift can come only from the mother, value is placed upon the uniqueness of breast feeding. As one mother said: 'It's something that no one else can have.' Another woman commented: 'It just seems you're closer to the baby if you breast feed and the baby's closer to you. I think it's an emotional thing, too, for you and the baby being close to each other. It makes your relationship with the child unique.'

The Decision to Breast Feed: How Was It Made?

Approximately half the women in the study arrived at the decision to breast feed as a result of a rational, considered analysis of the merits of breast feeding. They gathered information primarily from reading and talking with other women. A few women sought advice from their physicians. Others had learned of the value of breast feeding through educational or professional pursuits (e.g., during medical school, while working as a nurse). The majority of women reported making their decision during their pregnancy, although in other instances the decision had been made much earlier. For example, one woman decided she would breast feed when she was in Grade 8 after researching a paper on the pros and cons of breast feeding. Another decided to breast feed as a result of her course in paediatrics in medical school.

The other half of our study participants made reference to the fact that they did not make a decision to breast feed. It was simply taken for granted that they would always do so: 'I don't feel breast feeding was even a matter of decision. I always felt that was the way I wanted to do it and that was that.' / 'I always expected I would breast feed. I never even thought about it. I would have assumed you only would choose not to breast feed if for some reason you couldn't.' / 'I assumed I would breast feed. I didn't really sit and deliberate, will I or won't I.' Others saw it as a predictable accompaniment to having a baby: 'Breast feeding for me was really part of the whole process of having a child and not something that I really ever made a very conscious decision about.'

Cultural Influences on Breast Feeding

This acceptance of breast feeding, reflecting an unequivocal belief in its value, is striking given the relatively low incidence of breast feeding as recently as fifteen years ago. It suggests that many women have so completely internalized the newer beliefs on breast feeding that the alternate option of bottle feeding is deemed completely irrelevant. Only a few women commented that their decision to breast feed was influenced by what was happening around them. One woman, in reference to her choice to breast feed, said: 'You probably have to give credit to the times more than anything.' Another said: 'Years before I was even married when bottle feeding was more in vogue, I don't think I thought about breast feeding. Part of the interest has to be society, and the encouragement, and you start thinking about the bonding and the nutrients. At this point I'm not even considering bottle feeding unless there is a problem.'

The majority of women seemed oblivious to the idea that their attitudes might be shaped by the dominant culture. A few, however, recognized the subtle pressure that could be exerted:

They do a real guilt trip on people who don't breast feed. If I had decided not to breast feed I think I would be feeling the guilt.

I think quite honestly if I even mention that I think I'm going to bottle feed I'd get a lot of flak from everybody.

I still don't understand why I'm so determined to breast feed. There is that element of being a failure as a mother if I don't – that I'm giving her a second-class start in life. Actually I find even more pressure now than with the first child because the newspapers are full of articles – even our little neighbourhood paper.

The notion of second-class mothering was one that caused concern. One mother reflected:

My husband is not going to look down on me as being a bad mother if I don't breast feed. He's very understanding so I'm not pressured by him. I let myself be pressured by other people around me. I can't really differentiate between, 'Do I really want to do it or is it because people expect me to do it?' You hear about people complaining about sore nipples and being over-tired because it takes a lot out of you. So that makes me think, 'Are you sure you want to do that?' But then again if I don't do it I'm not a good mother. It's ambivalence.

An increase in breast-feeding rates is only one aspect of the many changes that have occurred in the last fifteen years in relation to maternity. The early pioneers of change struck a responsive chord in many women. Increasing numbers of women have fought against the mushrooming use of technology, which has threatened to strip them of their autonomy and dignity throughout pregnancy and delivery. Women have fought for and achieved more rights in decision making about birth options. They have resisted such things as fetal monitoring, Caesarian sections, and anaesthetized births. They have actively promoted breast feeding and have successfully pressed for changes in hospital policies to facilitate it. In general terms they have transformed the culture of maternity in a way that has positively benefited countless women. However, as cultural norms shift there is a cost to those whose attitudes and practices do not change accordingly. These people are out of step with the mainstream and risk being stigmatized because they do not conform to the dominant pattern. As we will see in the next chapter, women who decide to bottle feed feel this risk.

The majority of our study participants believed that it was incumbent upon mothers to provide what was 'best' for their children. In the perception of all the women in the study, breast feeding was, without doubt, the optimal choice for the baby. None the less, a few of the women recognized elements of dogmatism in the current culture of breast feeding. They were aware that breast feeding is often equated with 'proper mothering' and believed they would feel guilty if they chose to bottle feed or stop breast feeding early. While we enthusiastically promote breast feeding we must also bear in mind that other choices are not wrong but simply different. We must encourage women to make informed choices and then treat their decisions with respect.

CHAPTER FOUR

Choosing to Bottle Feed

The Decision to Bottle Feed

Many of the women we spoke to who intended to bottle feed discussed their decision in terms of personal choice. They felt pressured to breast feed but believed they must do what seemed right for themselves. Although breast feeding is clearly a desirable and healthy option, it is a choice that must be kept in perspective. In the industrialized countries of the world millions of infants have successfully survived on infant formula.

Women who opted to bottle feed were the ones who were most aware of the social pressures to breast feed. It was not an easy decision to make but a few women, after some soul searching, did just that. Louise described her point of view: 'These days breast feeding is sort of like the "in" thing to do and it's pushed at people. You're almost made to feel guilty if you don't breast feed because it's supposed to be such a great thing. But I don't think it's for everybody. I just feel that it's a matter of personal choice. I think you have to know yourself to make that choice and if you're just not that kind of person that can relax anywhere then breast feeding is not for you.'

Another woman initially assumed that she would breast feed. During her pregnancy she thought more seriously about it and realized she had not made this decision for herself. She explained: 'When I assumed I would breast feed, that decision didn't come from me at all. It was just from society, I think. Then I started thinking about it and I thought, "No, I don't have to, you know, I can do what I want." Just because your friends do it or people tell you to do it, you don't have to do it. If you're uncomfortable with it, don't do it.'

Carolyn, too, was aware of how influential societal pressure could be. When asked if there was anything she might say to other mothers that might help them in making a decision about bottle feeding, she responded: 'The only thing I can think is, "Just go with the way you really feel. Try not to be pressured by what you think everybody else is saying." Because I think there is a lot of that. I don't think the way you feed your baby dictates whether you're a good mother or a bad mother. It's what you feel and the care you give the child. If breast feeding doesn't work for you, cut it off. You find other ways of getting that bond with your baby. No one way is ever right for everybody.'

Some women reached their decision with little difficulty. Betty is a case in point: 'I've learned everybody's different. That's why when I decided to bottle feed, what everybody else said about breast feeding just didn't bother me a bit, because I know what I'm comfortable with. I'm looking at me, not everybody else.'

For others the decision was not so easy. Germaine discussed her feelings: 'It is hard to be the only one in a group of fifteen who has chosen to go one way. There is this suggestion, even on the cans of baby food, to tell you that breast milk is the preferred method. To make a decision to go against that you have to be fairly secure.' When asked if she felt guilty about her choice Germaine replied: 'Yes, mainly because of numbers. There's a great emphasis on breast feeding here. I know that it's by far the most popular method at the moment.' Lynnette, too, felt guilty: 'I am feeling guilty. Because I think, "Lynette, come on, this is better for the child." Then I think if I don't feel good about it, is it better for the child? I still have this nagging feeling that people will think, "Oh, she's not really a good mother." These days breast feeding is a cure-all for whatever ails you.'

In a feminist analysis of breast feeding Brack (1975) noted that in this pro-breast-feeding era women have no more control over their breasts than they did in the bottle-feeding era. Whenever women attempt to exert individual choices that run counter to dominant societal norms they are chastised and made to feel guilty.

Why Women Bottle Fed

Women bottle fed for a variety of reasons. A majority of the women we interviewed had tried breast feeding their first child and had run into problems. This confirmed the findings of an earlier study by Martin (1978) noting that feeding decisions made by mothers of more than one child were largely determined by their experience of feeding the previous child. They did not want a repetition of these difficulties. In other cases women believed bottle feeding would allow them more freedom. Women who bottle fed were usually uncomfortable with the idea of breast feeding in public and some placed a high priority on getting their figures back to normal as quickly as possible.

Women who reported previous difficulties with breast feeding described a range of problems. One woman, Sarah, had difficulties because she had inverted nipples. She was given one nipple shield in hospital but could not find any more like it when she returned home; she had to sterilize the one shield each time she fed. Engorgement posed additional problems. The baby's weight gain did not satisfy the doctor so he suggested formula. Sarah followed his advice and found it 'fantastic' and was also pleased her husband could participate in feeding.

Helen had bleeding nipples and no one to turn to for help. She was overwhelmed:

I had such sore bleeding nipples all the time, and I didn't know what to do. I was in such a panic 'cause I really felt strongly about breast feeding but I'd be sitting there nursing her, the tears would be rolling down my cheeks and I was gritting my teeth. I had ice packs and I didn't know what I was doing. I was just running around in circles. Then when I went to the doctor and the baby had lost weight from birth, I said, 'Forget it. If it's not doing the best for her, then who am I kidding?'

The demands of motherhood could come as a shock. Sometimes breast feeding was too much of an additional burden:

Breast feeding in itself, I think, is a very hard thing to do. In lots of ways, you feel like your soul is being drained out of you. There's such a big change just in having a baby. When you suddenly realize the baby's there and you're committed and there's no turning back. I think being tied in that way as well made breast feeding even harder. I would say that the emotional part was so negative that it made me decide the bottle will be better because if I'm happier that'll communicate to the baby and it'll make it better all the way around.

There were a few instances where women had breast fed their first child four to six months yet decided to bottle feed the second child. They wanted to make things as easy as possible for themselves and to avoid any experiences that might lead to unnecessary worry.

Some women decided to bottle feed from birth because they wanted the freedom they believed it would give them. They felt they could leave their babies in someone else's care without worrying about how or when they would be fed. Freedom also meant that the responsibility for feeding was less of a burden because it could be shared with others, especially the father.

The majority of the women who bottle fed were uncomfortable with the idea of breast feeding in public. This is consistent with other studies that found that women who bottle fed would be embarrassed breast feeding in public (Jones and Belsey 1977; Martin 1978). The women in this study were not necessarily opposed to public breast feeding but felt that they themselves could not do it: 'I just don't feel as open about showing my body in public although a lot of people do. I've got nothing against anybody else doing it, but for myself, I don't feel comfortable.' / 'I want to do things together as a family. You know, going to parks and things like that. If you're breast feeding you can't very well do that. Some women can go sit in the car and feed the baby. I couldn't do that. I'd be afraid someone might walk by and see me.'

If these women had chosen to breast feed they knew they would only feel comfortable feeding in private and they wished to avoid the social consequences of such a decision: 'Being at home and being with friends that you've known for years, sitting in front of them – breast feeding. Well, I just wouldn't. I would probably go to the bedroom or something like that. I still think it's a very private matter between mother and child.' / 'You feel funny leaving your company sitting there in the living room while you breast feed. Then kids wander in and it's kind of a private thing to me. I'm just not comfortable if anyone is there.'

Some of the women who chose to bottle feed did so primarily because of concerns about their appearance. They believed they could return to their pre-pregnancy shape more quickly if they bottle fed because they would not have to worry about drinking extra fluids or maintaining a special diet for breast feeding. Loni, a first-time mother, saw a film about breast feeding before her baby's birth. The film showed the body changes that accompany breast feeding such as larger breasts and nipples. Loni described her reaction: 'That really turned me off. I thought, "Oh, my God!" As soon as I have the baby, I want to get back to my normal shape as soon as possible. I wanted to start dieting and exercising. If you're breast feeding you can't really go on a stringent diet – you really have to watch what you eat and eat healthy food.' Unfortunately, after the baby was born Loni wanted to try breast feeding but her attempt failed because after the delivery she had taken medication to inhibit milk production. As a result of her brief experience with breast feeding she was determined to try again when she had her next child.

For a few others, weight loss was not an issue but dietary restrictions were: 'You can't eat onions. You can't take medication because it comes through in the milk, too. There's a lot of things you can't do when breast feeding.' / 'I think formula is pretty good, really. I doubt I have any good vitamins to really look after the baby. I'll eat the wrong stuff, you know; I just prefer the high calorie, greasy foods – hamburgers and things like that. I like to have french fries and maybe a nice bar of chocolate and then some coke and things like that.'

The influence of these women's husbands is of interest because, with one exception, they did not encourage their wives to bottle feed. Their attitudes ranged from indifference to a definite preference for breast feeding. Whatever their preference, the decision was always left up to the woman. Typical viewpoints of the husbands are illustrated by the following excerpts: 'My husband wanted me to breast feed. I guess it was just because it's best for your baby to breast feed. Finally, he didn't agree with me but he accepted my decision mainly because it was my body. He had no choice.' / 'Feeding is my decision, you know. He's the type that would try to help me no matter what. He's never questioned when I said that I would just go on the bottle this time.' A few of the women did note that their husbands enjoyed feeding the baby but this was not discussed as an important aspect of bottle feeding.

As we will see later in this book, these perceived obstacles to breast feeding need not be significant deterrents. Some of the obstacles have their roots in either misinformation or misconceptions about breast feeding. It is therefore important to ensure that women have access to accurate information. Some obstacles might have been overcome if women had more family or peer support. Other obstacles reflect certain societal realities. Although some forces in our culture encourage breast feeding there are others that act to discourage it. In later chapters we will see that breast feeding can be difficult, particularly if the mother is isolated. For some women, it adds too much of a burden during a time that is already full of challenges and changes to familiar patterns. Breast feeding can tie women to their homes. Some mothers do not mind; others chafe at it. We will see that it is not always easy or socially acceptable to breast feed in public. And in a culture that worships thinness and glorifies women's bodies as sex objects it is not surprising that some women have ambivalent feelings about the impact of breast feeding on their bodies. Women who make decisions that run counter to prevailing trends should not be judged harshly. Many of our attitudes and viewpoints are shaped by and reflect the influences of the world in which we live. They cannot always be easily discarded when new values emerge, especially when the social environment reinforces many of the old ones.

PART THREE

The Realities of Breast Feeding

This section of the book provides a comprehensive picture of breast feeding. It is based on the detailed descriptions provided by the women we interviewed and covers a broad range of experiences. It is *not* my intent to disparage breast feeding but to realistically document it so that women can prepare for it in a practical way. Margaret McCaffery wrote an editorial in the medical journal *Canadian Family Physician* following her experience of breast feeding. In reference to studies on duration of breast feeding she said: 'I can tell them why women stop breast feeding in four little words that infant feeding manuals never mention: it's damned hard work' (McCaffery 1984: 1441). In a humorous account, McCaffery, who was obviously highly informed and technically well prepared for breast feeding, described the trials and tribulations of nine months of it. She captured, in a nutshell, much of the content of this book. And, like most of our mothers, she concluded (p. 1442): 'At nine months, I think I can say with some conviction that breast feeding sometimes is a religious experience, but it's also hard work. Just because it's "natural" doesn't mean it's easy. But the alternatives? No thank you.' Realistic documentation of breast feeding is important. If women themselves and health professionals understand the nature of mothers' experiences we can work together to formulate and promote policies and programs that will better support breast feeding.

There are are frequent references throughout the text to the proportion of women who spoke about certain topics. These proportions have been included deliberately as a reminder that although this book documents a range of experiences on a given topic, some women did not fall within the range presented or did not discuss the topic with us. There are instances where a topic is presented in detail because some (but not all) women felt strongly about it. For example, the section in the next chapter on the physical discomforts of breast feeding implies that breast feeding can be an onerous thing to do. It is important to note, however, that only half the women we spoke to talked about the physical discomforts. Presumably, the half of our sample who did not discuss this topic did not find the discomforts sufficiently difficult to warrant talking about them. Nevertheless, it is important to present this topic because women need a realistic understanding of what *might* happen. Those who are in the midst of discomfort need to know that they are not alone and that there is not something uniquely wrong with them because they are finding this experience difficult.

Chapters 4 through 9 document the key features of breast feeding, including the physical discomforts, worry about the adequacy of one's breast milk, the variety of approaches to feeding schedules, the fatigue, the time commitments, and the challenges of breast feeding in public. These chapters illustrate the range of reactions women had and the stresses and strains they faced. It is human nature that we focus on the difficult aspects of our experiences and have less to say about the fine parts. Breast feeding is no exception. The women in our study, by virtue of the fact that they breast fed far longer than the average breast-feeding woman, clearly found their experience rewarding. The difficulties they encountered were not usually seen as reasons for stopping but as obstacles to be overcome. In the process of surmounting the problems they focused more on the difficulties than on the joys. Although many of the quotes hint at the pleasures of breast feeding, they are often overshadowed by the difficulties. Therefore, in chapter 10 the comments that reflect the rewards of breast feeding and the factors that made women want to continue are drawn together to convey the more positive aspects.

CHAPTER FIVE

The Physical Discomforts

The physical discomforts of breast feeding came as a surprise to a lot of women. Their image of a mother nursing peacefully in a rocking-chair bore little resemblance to some of the physical sensations and discomforts they experienced during the early weeks of breast feeding. About half our participants discussed the various discomforts, which included sore nipples, the feeling of the let-down reflex, leaking breasts, engorgement, and mastitis. Although discomfort alone did not deter women from continuing with breast feeding, it was a significant part of many women's experience.

Sore Nipples

Most women who spoke about physical discomforts complained of sore nipples, particularly during the early weeks of nursing. When the baby pulled on the nipple and fed frequently it caused soreness. Some women found that as the frequency of feeding decreased and the nipples toughened the pain subsided. Others had sensitive nipples for some time.

The degree of pain varied from mild to very severe. It was most severe just as the baby latched onto the nipple. One woman exclaimed, 'Just at the beginning, when he first starts to suck the pain is excruciating; it's unbelievable!' Another woman thought that her sore raw nipple 'was gonna fall off; it had a big crack in it.' A third woman found that her nipples felt like they were being bitten although the baby did not have any teeth: 'I've got sores all over the place and it's only been a couple of days. He feels like he's got twenty-five teeth in his mouth.'

The soreness could penetrate the whole breast, making it painful to even a slight touch. Often the pain was severe enough to demand special measures to counteract it:

I would do a breathing exercise from my pre-natal class. When the baby latched on I would count to ten and breathe really deeply because if I had gone 'Oh!' then the milk probably wouldn't come down and he'd sense that I'm tense. I would try and just breathe, calm down, and then by about ten seconds, he would have regulated it and it wouldn't hurt.

I find that when I have to start with the sore breast I dread the feed. One day on the weekend I was feeling guilty, feeling Alexander could feel my apprehension about this breast. He's just not taking it into his mouth as readily. So I try to divert my attention while he's feeding on it.

The nipple pain was emotionally as well as physically upsetting. One nursing mother had such severe pain that she began to dread breast feeding under any circumstances. After a period of soreness she said: 'I started to think that I didn't like the feeling of having her sucking on the nipples, *even* when they didn't hurt.' Another woman's feelings about breast feeding changed dramatically once the nipple pain had subsided: 'What a difference when your nipples aren't sore. It's amazing. It's a whole different experience.'

Nobody stopped breast feeding solely because of nipple pain. They all persevered. Some reminded themselves that the pain could not get worse: 'I was getting really cracked, sore nipples. My concern was how much sorer can they get? How am I going to be able to keep up with it? The soreness bothered me but I kept thinking how much worse can it get.' / 'I figure it'll get better as time goes by so I'll persevere.' The perceived benefit to the baby was an important motivator for continuing to breast feed despite the pain: 'The third day I said, "It's so sore now I can't stand it." Yet I was doing it because I wanted her to have it.'

Women tried a number of approaches to prevent the pain. Dry, cracked, or raw nipples were treated with mineral oil or lanolin-based creams. Exposing the nipples to air was the most frequently mentioned pain remedy. As one woman explained: 'At night I try to sleep with my nipples exposed. After four hours of that it's not as bad. At the end of the day if I haven't run around with my nipples exposed, it's really quite painful by the late evening feeding.' Women also tried nipple shields, altering breast-feeding positions, occasional bottle feeding, and nipple massage as ways of coping with or adapting to nipple pain.

Let-down and Leaking

When oxytocin is released into the mother's bloodstream, milk is released in the breast from alveoli, ducts, and the sinuses towards the nipple. The milk is then readily available to the baby when he or she suckles. If this release of milk, called the let-down reflex, is strong enough, the nursing woman's breasts leak without the stimulation of suckling.

Of the women interviewed, less than one-third discussed the let-down reflex. Of these, most could feel when let-down occurred. When the let-down sensation was mild, women talked about it in terms of a tingling 'pins and needles' feeling. When the let-down sensation was strong it was painful. Women did not talk at length about milk let-down sensations. Painful let-down, however, was described in vivid terms: 'It's kind of like somebody's holding a muscle real tight while you're pushing against it. It feels like the milk's coming in. It's like a small engorgement every time.' / 'It's like knives right through my breast. It's a "grit your teeth" type of feeling for a good thirty seconds. Once the milk starts flowing it's still uncomfortable but not unpleasant.'

Some women noticed that the let-down occurred when any baby cried in the early weeks. In time, their bodies became more selective in responding to their own baby's cry. For some, even that response diminished and let-down occurred only after the baby suckled. The changes in the pattern of let-down are evident in the following excerpt:

At the beginning it was terrible. My let-down didn't know where to let down. I had Larry's entire family here one day and he had beers out in the garden. I'm not usually a beer drinker but I drank it because it's supposed to create milk. I didn't realize it was creating milk. I was wearing a white shirt and it was just drenched. Now, nothing like that happens. It's amazing how attuned it becomes to your baby's cry. First it was just the wheels on the buses outside that would make me let down.

During the day I would have a tingly feeling two or three times when I know my milk would be there. Then it would subside. I don't have that anymore and when he nurses he has to bring the milk down. Before the milk always was there when he was ready but now he has to suck for about ten seconds. He'll stop and look up at me. There'll be nothing. He'll come back for about another five seconds and then I can feel it come down.

Women who felt the let-down were certain they had milk. Conversely, when they could not, they were less confident that they were producing milk. Incorrectly, some women correlated milk supply and the let-down: 'When the hour mark would come, even if he wasn't crying, I could feel the milk letting down. I could feel tingling in my breasts. It was a great feeling that, "Boy, this is really working."' / 'In the last couple of weeks I just really felt I wasn't producing a lot of milk. That feeling of let-down has not been there as much and when I've gone long stretches without nursing I haven't felt myself filling up or anything like that.'

When let-down resulted in leaking breasts women were much more vocal. Almost half the nursing women in our study discussed leaking breasts. Most found them annoying. Many were embarrassed if their wet clothes were obvious to others. They disliked waking up in wet and sticky beds. For some, leaking breasts was one of the worst aspects of breast feeding. One woman, for instance, said: 'The only thing I couldn't stand is my breasts leaking. It used to drive me crazy.' Other women shared their feelings:

You feel very motherly and the next minute you think, 'I am a cow. Look at it! It's just gushing.' I would wake up in pools of milk the first month. After sleeping all night the breasts would have leaked. All this milk would be in the sheets and it was so wet and sticky and gooey.

I used to cry when I used to leak a lot in bed. This was before she slept through. I used to suddenly cry and feel like I was a cow or something.

It can be very messy. As soon as the baby starts crying they start dripping. You get milk all over everywhere and that's quite annoying. I'm sitting drenched in milk.

Sheila Kitzinger, a British childbirth educator and social anthropologist, speculated about why women have such strong negative reactions to leaking in her book *The Experience of Breast Feeding* (1979). She noted that many women think of breast milk as an unclean secretion that streams out unbidden at inconvenient times. She links these feelings to the difficulties of integrating the radical shift in the mental image of a woman's body at the time of pregnancy and birth. She described these marked changes (pp. 206–7):

At one moment it is full and ripe with child, and at the next it is empty and open. At one moment she is two people, one tucked inside the other; at the next she is a mother having to relate to a strange little creature who is handed to her squashed and crying. Before birth her body is closed, its boundaries containing her baby. After birth it is sagging and leaking, the surface damp and sweating, the perineum sore, orifices stretched, tissues bruised and tender, with sticky liquids, it seems, dripping from every opening.

It is no wonder, she says, that women feel ambivalent because they equate leaking with other body fluids like sweat, pus, or nasal mucous, all of which are discharged involuntarily. This would be especially true for those who feel shame at exposing a part of the body that is normally conceived of as sexual and kept hidden.

At a practical level, leaking was simply an irritant; women tired of the damp, sticky feeling and the extra efforts to cope with the smell and the soiled clothes:

I leak more at night than in the daytime when I've got the bra on. I'm not going to wear the bra at night because it's uncomfortable. I have face-cloths that I put across my breasts so I'm not sleeping in a totally wet bed. It makes wet spots anyway because the face-cloths move. They're damp and uncomfortable in the morning and feel messy. It doesn't feel sticky on your body. It's all psychological. You just know you have liquid all over you all night. You feel you need a shower. I just get tired of that and of having to put kleenexes or whatever into my bra and of having to wear a bra.

That's one problem, the fact that your clothes get filled with milk all over the place. It doesn't stain. It's just that after a while you get this dried milk smell that's not exactly pleasant.

My leaking breasts are getting me down. I feel like I always need a shower. I've got about six blouses that I wash each day and I'm going through three bras a day so it's a lot of work. I feel like I'm never very presentable. So it is a major problem.

Women found obvious wet spots on their clothes embarrassing. Fern related an experience that was common to others: 'Last week I was out and I got way behind. I just started to leak and my whole shirt was soaked. It was sort of embarrassing because I'm walking down the street and everybody's looking at me. I can't really cover up this shirt that's soaked. Some of the women sort of smile to themselves because they knew what was happening but the men were looking. It was embarrassing.'

Although mothers talked about the embarrassment and irritation associated with leaking, it did not deter them from going out. They became adept at choosing clothing that would disguise the presence of leaked milk and many used breast pads. Most disliked wearing bras with inserted pads and almost all objected to the cost of disposable pads. Some experimented with washable bra inserts or home-made pads. Most women discovered there were no other options: 'I find breast pads are a pain in the butt because you can see them through just about everything you wear. It's so annoying. It's frustrating to try to decide what I can wear when I go outside. You know everyone's going to see these breast pads, but I don't really know quite how to get around it. I need them because I am a leaker.'

The women who discussed leaking had not realized in advance that it would be such a problem. Two women speculated on its potential impact: 'I could see how some women could give it up because you're constantly wet.' / 'If leaking had been a big problem where you couldn't get dressed or were leaking all the time, it could be embarrassing. You might start to have negative feelings after a certain amount of time.' Others felt differently. One woman decided that after a while 'you get kind of cavalier about it' and another said you learned to cope: 'You become a pro.'

Engorgement

Few women talked about engorgement. Those who did generally became engorged when their milk first came in or when the baby slept longer than expected and a feeding was missed. Engorgement was very painful for some women. Karla found that she became so preoccupied with the pain that she was unable to think clearly about what could be causing it or how she could relieve it:

One night I got totally engorged and the pain – pain like you wouldn't believe! Stupid me – I don't know where my brain was, but I didn't realize I was engorged. I was in pain and I thought, 'Oh, I've got a breast infection.' I said, 'Norm, I'm sure it's cancer, they're gonna have to cut it off.' I was in such pain I couldn't even think. I was putting my breast in a bowl of hot water. I had a shower then about 3:30 in morning. I thought, 'Karla, pump your breast.' It was just terrific and I thought, 'You're so stupid.' I was so caught up with the pain, never having had it.

Another woman had problems with engorgement in one breast because her baby occasionally would nurse on only one side. She endured the pain for fear of encouraging more milk production if she pumped: 'There were times when she would go five hours and then I would wake her because I was uncomfortable and she would only nurse on one side and go right back to sleep. The other poor side would go eight hours. I was afraid to express it thinking I would just encourage more to come in.'

Women dealt with engorgement in a number of ways. Hot compresses, hot showers, and massages were used to stimulate the let-down and facilitate pumping. Others woke their babies and fed them.

Mastitis

Mastitis is a condition characterized by a red, swollen, hot, and painful area on the breast accompanied by flu-like symptoms in the mother. It results from untreated plugged ducts and differs from this condition only in degree. Women had difficulty differentiating between a blocked duct and mastitis: 'I all of a sudden woke up with it one morning. The whole side

The Physical Discomforts 43

of me just felt terrible. At first it felt like I had a bit of a fever and mastitis. It turned out it was just a blocked duct.' / 'I just got feeling really draggy. Just pushing along all day. I was a little bit sore, but I didn't really realize what it was until later. I took my temperature, then I realized what it was.' Because of the similarity of the symptoms this confusion is not surprising.

Steph's experience illustrates the nature of mastitis. She was interviewed in the middle of a breast infection. Her concern over her condition is apparent in the detail with which she described her experience. Steph had felt miserable. For two days she had noticed pain and redness around her nipple. She then discovered she had a fever: 'I told my doctor that I'd been having a 102° temperature at the time. It had gone from 98.8° to 102° in three hours. I just couldn't do anything. My husband came home, checked my temperature and by 7:30 I was just miserable.' Steph remembered reading about mastitis and went back to the books to confirm the symptoms. Once confirmed, she speculated about the causes: 'I hadn't been putting any lotion on. That's probably how I cracked it. So it got infected.' The doctor prescribed antibiotics and recommended that she express milk from the infected breast rather than nurse.

Steph's husband cared for the baby while she had mastitis but she could not escape some activites: 'The baby wants to stay up [to] around 11:00. That was difficult because of mastitis. My husband was trying to get him to go to sleep, but it wasn't working. I said, "Let me get up." After I had the penicillin I got worse. I got the shakes really bad, my teeth were chattering, and my fever was really high. I finally got up at 11:00 because my husband was having no luck with the baby. I rocked him in the chair and fed him and he went to sleep.' That night her fever broke and she got a six-hour sleep before waking up with a pounding headache. At the time of the interview Steph was still slightly feverish and her breast was sore. She said it felt engorged, 'but it's different, more pain, and sometimes the pain is sharp and my breast is very hot.' She found that expressing milk from the sore breast relieved the pain.

A variety of emotions welled to the surface during this period. Steph was annoyed with herself over her lack of nipple care. She felt guilty about not nursing from both breasts while she had mastitis. She was also overwhelmed by the discomfort to the point that she cried because she 'was feeling so terrible with pain.' However, once the infection healed Steph and her baby had no trouble re-establishing nursing.

The discomforts described in this chapter were irritating, but for the most part they were viewed as nothing more than a nuisance. As we will see in chapter 12, it was only when these discomforts were added to a number of other irritations that they became a key factor in a decision to stop breast feeding.

CHAPTER SIX

Assessing the Milk Supply

The adequacy of the supply of breast milk was an issue with many women in this study. Attention first focused on supply when the milk initially 'came in,' an event that marked the beginning of 'real' nursing. Women then applied a variety of criteria to assess the adequacy of their supply. Those who lacked confidence in breast feeding often used inappropriate criteria to judge their milk supply and so incorrectly assumed they had insufficient milk. A few women who thought their supply was good found their confidence undermined by advice given by physicians. Over one-third of the women interviewed talked about supply.

Although some women spoke of concern about their milk supply, it was neither a major issue in the study nor a primary factor in early cessation of breast feeding. By contrast, concerns about milk supply feature prominently in the professional literature on breast feeding (Florack et al. 1984; Greiner, Van Esterik, and Latham 1981; Gussler and Briesemeister 1980; Simopoulos and Grave 1984; Tully and Dewey 1985; Whichelow 1982; World Health Organization 1981). These major studies and reviews on duration of breast feeding emphasize insufficient milk as a primary reason why women stop breast feeding prematurely. So much attention and controversy has surrounded this topic that it has been given the label insufficient milk syndrome (IMS for short).

There has been a good deal of discussion about the causes of IMS. Some authors have suggested that negative emotional attitudes towards breast feeding can actually result in a physical inability to nurse (Bentovim 1976; Sears, Maccoby, and Levin 1957). Greiner et al. (1981) believe that the best explanation for IMS is the impact of supplemental formula feedings on milk production. Others have suggested that mothers simply use the category 'insufficient milk,' which they view as a culturally acceptable rationalization, to justify a decision to stop breast feeding that may have been made for other less socially acceptable reasons (Gussler and Briesemeister 1980).

When the Milk Comes In

Soon after delivery, in response to the stimulus of suckling and a change in hormone levels, mature milk was produced. Women noticed that milk had replaced colostrum when their breasts felt full or when they expressed white milk rather than yellow colostrum. When milk replaced colostrum women believed that their milk had 'come in.'

The presence of milk, as opposed to 'just colostrum,' was ascribed considerable importance. Women knew that colostrum delivered antibodies to the infant, yet they believed nursing had not begun until the milk arrived. They felt pride, wonder, and joy when their milk came in:

I felt really proud the first night I realized that my breasts were becoming engorged. I realized that they were becoming a little hard and a little sore and I thought, 'Oh, it's working.' It was nice. It was uncomfortable, but I just felt so proud of it.

When the milk came in, it was marvellous. I can't explain it because the breast is symbolic of different things. It's thinking, 'This is what it's really for, not a sexual thing.' When you feel a prickly feeling that the milk is coming down you constantly feel that your body's working to look after this child. I find anything like that quite incredible. I can't explain it really other than it was quite interesting and exciting. 'Now I have something to give you because before it was just the colostrum!' That's the beginning of the whole nursing, when the milk comes in and you just start.

Some women said their milk came in gradually. They did not experience engorgement or fullness of their breasts or feelings of let-down. Others worried about whether their milk had come in at all. Doubts were quelled when mothers were told that their infants were emptying the breast before it had a chance to fill with milk to the point of discomfort. Expressing some milk from the breast so that the mother could see it also relieved doubts.

Indicators of Adequate Supply

Once the milk came in many women turned their attention to the adequacy of their milk supply and worried that they would not have enough milk to nourish their babies. They used a variety of criteria to decide if they had enough milk.

Breast fullness was used initially as an indicator of the presence of milk: 'I've got tons of milk. My breasts are really big and lumpy. There's lots of milk in them now. I'm sure I've got lots of milk all the time.' After several weeks the breasts became softer so this marker was no longer useful.

Women were reassured when they saw milk spurt from the breast. This often happened in the bath or shower as hot water stimulated milk flow or if the baby suddenly pulled away from the breast during nursing: 'He's nursed sometimes a good half hour, forty minutes, and I've checked to make sure there's milk there and there is. It's squirting all over the place. I'll pull him off and it's beaned him in the face and all over. Or else he gets off the breast and I'll be looking around and I look down and the poor kid's drenched his face. It's squirting so there's milk. Somehow I'm productive.' Some women noticed that occasionally their milk came down so quickly from the breast that it seemed to choke the baby: 'He'll start at the breast and get it going. Then he'll start to choke and pull off. It comes out in a little spurt. So one thing I haven't had any difficulty with at all is milk supply.'

When the baby was content after feeding, mothers assumed their supply was adequate: 'My milk supply has increased to meet his demands and I've had no problems. It's amazing how it can increase and decrease. He seems to be satisfied with what he's getting. It's not like he's crying afterwards.' Likewise, if the baby was thriving, it was obvious that everything was in order: 'I definitely had enough milk to feed her. She was definitely gaining and doing well.' / 'She's got to be getting more than enough. I can't weigh her but I can tell just by looking at her she's not starved.'

Low Supply: What To Do?

Women who reported confidence in breast feeding could objectively assess why they might have a poor supply. They knew that fatigue, anxiety, and a low fluid intake were important factors in a decreased supply. The following excerpts are typical of women's comments about fluctuations in supply:

The night of the christening I had to supplement her. I ran out. I wasn't totally surprised 'cause I'd been doing a lot of running around for a couple of days prior.

Over Christmas my milk supply was low because I was doing too much for the last week.

My milk supply seems to be so sensitive to anxiety. I really wasn't worried about this last set of exams but my milk went way down. When I had my paediatrics oral I talked to the paediatricians. They said anxiety and fatigue are two really big things to make your milk supply go down. That night I noticed she was getting more. The next day it just seemed that she was getting gallons.

They also knew how to improve the situation: 'Last Thursday and Friday I thought, "I'm gonna take it easy, stay in bed, try to do what the books say." If you feel you're not supplying enough for the baby you have to stop and relax.'

Women took more care to ensure that their food and fluid intakes were adequate and they fed more frequently. They understood the supply and demand principle of breast feeding: the more the infant suckled, the more milk they would have. The results were usually quite obvious: 'I've proved it to myself that just by more feeding and forcing her to have more, I've increased the supply. In fact, it's really going to waste because I can't feed her as much as I'd like to. I mean I can't wake her up all the time.' Those women who knew that their supply was bound to undergo fluctuations could respond to changes by eliminating possible causes. At the same time, there were women who lacked confidence in breast feeding and therefore found it difficult to assess the situation objectively. These women were frequently haunted by worries about the adequacy of their milk.

With bottle feeding, mothers rely on visual standards to measure the adequacy of their baby's consumption. There is less need to judge intake by assessing such things as the baby's satisfaction or the number of wet diapers. Because we are accustomed to thinking in terms of number of ounces consumed it is difficult for some women to trust what cannot be measured. Almost half the women who discussed supply mentioned doubts about whether they had enough milk. They worried because they could not see how much the baby had drunk. As they speculated about the adequacy of their milk they focused on indicators that did not accurately reflect an adequate supply, e.g., soft breasts, a fussy baby, frequent feedings. Ironically, they often ignored other criteria such as wet diapers and adequate growth that would have indicated an adequate supply.

When the milk initially comes in, the breasts become full because of glandular changes and increased blood circulation. Once the milk production becomes established the breasts feel soft even though they are producing copious amounts of milk. Unfortunately, this softness was interpreted by some women as indicating they had an insufficient amount of milk. Many women talked about their soft breasts. The next two quotes are typical:

The thing about breast feeding is not knowing whether he's had enough. In the beginning, your breasts get full and you know you've got a lot of milk. After you've been feeding for awhile they don't get as full. It's only when you miss a feed and start filling up you know you've got lots of milk. Otherwise you've got this feeling of uneasiness about how much the baby has actually had.

I find within that period when the baby is feeding every two to two and a half hours in the evening my breasts don't really seem to replenish themselves. They seem very soft. It becomes an endless thing. He doesn't seem to be very satisfied by the second feeding. He seems to be much more satisfied if I let the breast get firmer. I know it's not supposed to work that way, that the more frequently the baby sucks is supposed to make your breasts replenish themselves. It doesn't seem to work that way for me.

Doubts about supply were fuelled when a baby was not content during or just after feeding. It was difficult for women to dissociate the feeding from the baby's distress: 'I get concerned when Mick cries after I breast feed wondering whether he has enough or if I should keep feeding him longer.' / 'When the baby is crying after a feeding you think he's crying because he's not getting anything to eat. You think you haven't got enough milk.'

A baby's sleeplessness was also viewed as a sign of discontent, which, in turn, contributed to anxiety in some women: 'When the baby never slept I thought she wasn't sleeping because she wasn't getting enough. My mother tended to feed into that a lot. So I had a bit of a crisis with the breast feeding because I started to think I was starving her.' Babies cry for a variety of reasons and crying during or after nursing is not necessarily indicative of inadequate milk. These babies may have needed cuddling, a diaper change, or burping, or may simply have had fussy temperaments.

Many women were unprepared for the frequent feedings that are part of breast feeding. Some women believed their breast-fed babies should not want to nurse any more frequently than every three to four hours. They were distressed to discover that their baby sometimes wanted to be fed as frequently as every half-hour to two hours. These mothers began to doubt their supply when the baby's demands were inconsistent with their expectations: 'The erratic timing of her feeding makes you feel as though she wants it so desperately. You question, what are you doing wrong that you can't get her to get milk?' / 'I'm concerned whether my milk is rich enough. The fact that she's eating so often makes me feel sometimes as if she's not really satisfied.'

It is well documented that many breast-fed babies nurse frequently. Bottle feeding standards of three to four hours between feedings are not always applicable to the breast-fed baby, yet this is still the standard many breast-feeding women use. Although most women in this study had learned from reading, pre-natal classes, and other nursing women that breast-fed babies nurse more frequently, they were still confused when it happened to them. Knowledge about this topic was not necessarily enough to allay anxieties, especially if other people implied that frequent nursing indicates a problem.

Fuelling Doubt: Physicians

There were a few situations where women's doubts about the adequacy of their milk supply were fuelled by comments of physicians. Physicians are generally viewed as experts on health matters and so hold considerable power of influence. Even when a woman disagreed with a physician's assessment it was difficult for her to trust that her own interpretation was correct.

Fiona, for example, noticed her baby was unusually fussy shortly after nursing. She called her paediatrician to ask what he thought might be causing the baby's changed behaviour. When he heard Fiona was breast feeding he immediately suggested the baby's fussiness was due to insufficient milk and recommended a formula supplement. Fiona recalled her reaction:

I got really upset about it. But he said he wanted to see Alexander in his office and we took him down. He saw the baby and said, 'He seems perfectly healthy.' Then he said, 'Your baby's basically starving to death.' I got really upset. He suggested, 'Go out and get some formula and still feed him with the breast and if he's hungry in between the breast give him formula and see if that works over the weekend. See if that calms him down and that way we'll know if he's hungry or not.'

Although she had mixed feelings about giving formula Fiona followed the doctor's advice. During this time, Fiona was experiencing breast pain, but in the confusion of the visit had forgotten to mention it to the doctor. Shortly after the appointment she noticed a sore on her breast that was oozing and bleeding. She called the La Leche League, learned that it was an abscess, and stopped nursing from that breast. She described her course of action: 'I've been frantically trying to reach my obstetrician thinking, "Well, I better get this breast treated so I can start feeding soon." And in the meantime, every three hours I've been expressing the milk out of the bad breast so it doesn't become engorged. Each time I express seven ounces of milk out of that one breast. That makes me feel good.'

Seeing so much milk reassured Fiona. She had believed all along that she had enough milk but the paediatrician's comments made her doubt it. The issue of adequate milk supply can have strong emotional overtones, as Fiona's comments illustrate: 'When I was at that paediatrician's office on Saturday I felt like a very incompetent female. I felt guilty as a mother. I felt all kinds of negative feelings.' The concrete

Assessing the Milk Supply 53

evidence of the expressed milk restored Fiona's confidence. She called the paediatrician to let him know about her success in expressing milk and to set the record straight about her milk supply:

So I feel good. I felt like, well, that guy's kind of full of shit because I do know I have milk. I called him back and I told him and he said, 'Okay, well, that does answer our question.' 'It did make sense,' he said, 'because when there's an abscess and when there's infection some of the ducts can get blocked and the baby may not have been getting enough milk.' I was willing to concede to that, to say, 'Okay, then we were both right. You know I'm not starving my child but you're right, the formula's needed right now to top up until I can get the breast back together.'

If the paediatrician had taken the time to question Fiona about the circumstances surrounding the baby's unusual fussiness the crisis of confidence could have been avoided. As it happened, Fiona's breast abscess was a mixed blessing because she at least discovered her milk supply was adequate.

Laurie also had an upsetting experience with her paediatrician. She had noticed her baby's feeding habits had changed in the week prior to her appointment with the paediatrician. The baby was now demanding to be fed every two hours. Feedings had been less frequent before. Laurie thought the increased frequency of nursing indicated the baby was going through a growth spurt and asked the paediatrician what he thought. She was surprised at his answer: 'He said, "Well, you don't have enough milk. He's at least a pound underweight. He should weigh at least nine pounds by now and he only weighs eight pounds. I'm pretty sure the reason is because he's just not getting enough. You know it's not very pleasant for a baby to suck on an empty breast." I was really taken aback by this.'

The paediatrician recommended a formula supplement and explained how to prepare it. When he finished giving instructions, he turned his back to Laurie and the baby and began to write on the charts. Laurie shared her feelings about this interaction: 'It was kind of upsetting and I had to get the baby dressed again and he was crying and the doctor just sat there with his back turned to me and I felt rather stupid and inept and I felt guilty. I thought, "Oh, my God, no wonder this poor kid has been feeding so frequently and crying and demanding to be fed and so on." I was very, very upset.'

When Laurie arrived home she reread her breast-feeding books and decided not to introduce formula because 'that is the beginning of the end and then you stop increasing your own milk supply.' Laurie admitted she was 'very teary' as she tried to assess what to do. She thought about why her milk supply might be low: 'I also decided in thinking about the week, what a stupid week it had been because that was the week I'd spent a day at the office and missed two feedings and I'd been out and I'd been driving around and going to visit friends and not napping and not drinking enough liquids and it had also been extremely hot.' Laurie tried to increase her milk supply by increasing her fluid intake. She made a concerted effort to rest and pumped milk from her breasts. She soon concluded that she had solved her problem.

Laurie was disappointed that her paediatrician was so ready to suggest switching to formula instead of giving advice on how to increase her supply. She described her reaction: 'Well, it really was upsetting. It was one thing to hear it from a mother or a mother-in-law where you can easily discount it but it's another thing to hear it from a paediatrician who supposedly supports breast feeding. But he certainly didn't. He didn't talk to me about any methods of increasing my milk supply. I was just appalled and I was just disgusted.'

Perhaps the paediatrician did not think to offer constructive support for breast feeding because he did not believe that breast milk was necessary for a healthy baby. He was no doubt unaware of how much Laurie needed and wanted support for breast feeding. She commented on what she believed the paediatrician should have been concerned about: 'As guilty as he made me feel, he made me feel guilty for the wrong reasons. I probably should have felt more guilty about not taking better care of *myself* and not thinking more about what was going on.' Laurie went on to explain that despite the emotional upset resulting from the paediatrician's assessment his advice at least encouraged her to assess the situation:

The paediatrician was a catalyst. He made me go out and talk to other people and do more reading and so on. It turned out for the best. It was not anything to do with exactly what he said and certainly not the way he said things, but at least it got me to do something that I should have really been doing, which is just staying home more and relaxing more and drinking more and really thinking about my milk supply not in an anxious way, not sitting back and wondering if I have enough milk, but in a very proactive way, doing something to make sure that I have enough.

In the cases of both Fiona and Laurie, the physician's comments led the mothers to question their activities, but not their ability to produce adequate milk supplies. They understood the nature of breast feeding sufficiently and resisted the advice. As we will see in chapter 13, Laurie's confidence did not stand the test of time. Both incidents had an emotional cost that could have been avoided if the physician had discussed the situation in detail and helped the mother examine alternatives to supplementation.

Women described how their feelings of being adequate mothers were linked to their abilities to nurse successfully. Both Fiona and Laurie thought they had failed as mothers because they were not providing enough milk. Other women also shared this sentiment: 'Your ability to breast feed is really tied up with your feelings of adequacy as a mother. It's really depressing because you think, "Oh, there's something wrong with me and I'm not really cut out to do this."' / 'Because of the frustration in feeding I felt very inadequate as a mother.' / 'It's funny how much your self-approval is all tied up with how much milk you've got.' Feelings of inadequacy and frustration could themselves contribute to a decrease in milk supply and aggravate existing supply problems. It must become a priority of physicians who deal with breast-feeding women to offer them moral support.

CHAPTER SEVEN

Feeding Schedules

There are two general approaches to handling feedings. In scheduled feeding the mother controls when the baby eats by offering the breast only at regular intervals, thus establishing a schedule. In demand feeding the baby sets his or her own feeding times. Over two-thirds of the women talked about feeding schedules. Half of these fed on a schedule and half fed on demand.

Schedule Feeding

The hospital was one source of pressure to feed on a schedule. Although doctors and nurses did not openly encourage schedule feeding it was implicit in other recommendations. Women were told to nurse no more frequently than every two hours, no less frequently than four or five. Unless the baby was 'rooming in' he or she was brought to the mother every four hours.

It came as a shock to some women that the baby didn't fall into that pattern at home: 'Within a three-hour period he's usually back on the breast one time. In the first few days I was allowing that to bother me because I was getting hung up with the hospital saying the time between feedings shouldn't be longer than four hours, or shorter than two hours.' / 'This schedule is quite different from the one at the hospital. So he's a little bit mixed up and I'm a little bit mixed up.'

There were isolated reports of other sources of pressure to schedule feed. One woman, who schedule fed her baby and liked routine in her life, believed that there was pressure from society at large to establish a schedule. She explained: 'You still want to be able to have some kind of routine to your life because it's so upset when you come home with the baby. You want to have something that you can say: she's every three hours or four hours. Society expects that you have the baby on some kind of a routine. Even though you believe strongly in breast feeding, somehow you still like some kind of routine you can count on.'

Another woman found that her neighbours had unsolicited advice to offer on the matter of feeding times: 'My next door neighbours were telling me, "Oh my goodness, he should be on a schedule now, he's ten weeks old. There should be a schedule set out by six weeks." They scheduled their children. It didn't matter what came along. It was necessary to feed at 9, 1, 5, 9, 1, 5. After you do this for a few weeks the baby falls into it.'

Family members, particularly mothers-in-law, were most frequently mentioned as a source of pressure. The following excerpt is from a woman who had both her mother-in-law and husband encouraging her to schedule feed:

That was the big thing – a schedule. My mother-in-law was a deep believer in scheduling. So is my husband. They kept saying, 'You should put her on a schedule.' They finally convinced me that we should try something because I was nursing her all the time. They did have a point. I see it now – it was a good thing to do because if she ate on a schedule she ate every four or three hours. She'd get a full tummy and she'd eat her next meal, and she'd have a good break in between feedings. The other way she'd be snacking every hour, hour and a half. It was hard on me because I never really knew when she wanted to eat. So I went along with that for a little while. I don't know how we did it, but she did do it. She ate every four hours. The hour she fed was messed up, depending on what time she woke up in the morning. I didn't mind that but it bothered my husband. He didn't like it if I had to feed her right at supper time or lunch time. He wanted it more routine; he's a real routine person. But it worked itself out. He got over that.

Some women chose to schedule feed simply because they wanted to. They spoke of the advantages of not feeling they were at the baby's 'beck and call.' They wanted to know that they would have certain times of the day to do things for themselves or with others. The following excerpts, from women who believed in schedule feeding, make reference to issues of control, freedom, and the importance of a pattern:

You have to discipline them a little bit and get them into a routine. Otherwise they'd just wake up whenever they feel like it.

To me a schedule is everything. It means I can get out of the house and my husband can give him the bottle.

Breast feeding just seemed to go on and on and you try to get him settled and he wouldn't sleep. Then you were on to the next feeding. So you were into the same cycle all over again. I wasn't rigid about a four-hour schedule but I tried to keep him on some sort of schedule because I felt I had to have some control over it. Otherwise he would be feeding all the time.

Other women talked about how schedule feeding helped them maintain peace of mind: 'It's nice to have some kind of pattern to your day, just for your own sanity.'
Schedule feeding did not necessarily work perfectly and most women compromised. Babies were not always hungry at feeding time and were sometimes hungry between feedings. The following excerpt is typical of the comments of many women: 'My own schedule is out of whack. I'm the type of person for whom 12 o'clock is lunch and you go to bed at 1 o'clock. You're trying to get these things on schedule

but you can't. How do you tell a baby it's not feeding time yet?'

Women occasionally gave in completely and adapted the schedule to suit their babies. The following two excerpts are from a woman who found she had to make a schedule adjustment in order to have a happier baby. She described her first approach:

My friends and husband were giving me a hard time saying that my milk was too weak or not enough because she's still sucking her thumb. I said, 'This is it!' I know she's getting enough. She's going to have to stick to either a three- or four-hour schedule. So all I do is get her up, play some music, and just rock her till she goes to sleep. If she's really really bad, I give her a bit of water. Then I put her back, and I have a rule – I let her cry for fifteen minutes. If she's still crying, then I get her up and just hug her.

After a week of this Daisey made some changes: 'She's been crying an awful lot. You don't know what to do. I finally decided rather than put her on four-hour feeds, I would put her on three-hour feeds and now I'm trying to feed her on demand. It seems to be working out much better.'

Demand Feeding

The women who found the regimentation of schedule feeding difficult decided to demand feed. Some, like Daisey, had tried schedule feeding and found it did not work for them. Others believed it was unrealistic to expect babies to follow a routine. These women were not able to keep a schedule themselves and did not expect their babies to follow one either:

I don't think you can regiment their lives at this point. I really don't think you can program them. They have such minds of their own that they decide this is the way they want things. Provided it's not detrimental to anyone's health or well being, then why not?

I never work on schedules including when I'm working. I would never have that expectation for my kid even though I would like him to be that way because it would make my life easier. My expectation would be that I would never be able to predict when he'd want to eat. It would never occur to me to put the baby on a schedule because this is much easier.

Other women emphasized the variability among babies and the need to respond to each baby individually.

Women who demand fed saw advantages to this method of feeding. Because the baby was fed when hungry, he or she was more contented. Overall, this made life less taxing. As well, the baby's frequent feedings (as is common with demand feeding) reduced the risk of breast discomfort due to full breasts.

Like schedule feeding, demand feeding also had its drawbacks. The major one was the unpredictability of feeding times. Some women adjusted easily to the variable feeding times. As one woman explained, it was 'just a matter of not being able to tell people what time I'd be able to do anything.' Others were not so relaxed. One mother said the unpredictability was driving her crazy. Another lost confidence in her milk supply because feedings were erratic; she introduced formula.

Women who demand fed found, as the schedule feeders predicted, that they were controlled by their babies. One mother described an episode with her two-month-old that illustrates the impact: 'I took him out for a carriage ride. He cried the whole time. I knew it was because he wanted to be on the breast. I brought him home, put him on the breast, and he fed for another half hour. He'd just been feeding for an hour before I took him out. I put him in the carriage, and we started over again.' This woman also expressed frustration over not being able to get anything done because of the constant demands of feeding: 'I don't think he should be nursing for the next few months on the same kind of routine that he has now, which is nursing all day. We don't get anything done. We don't do anything. I don't mind sitting here and feeding him and playing with him. I'll do that day in and day out. I'm putting a lot of faith in demand feeding. He really does control when he eats.'

After some period of adaptation, women usually stayed with one type of feeding schedule.

Frequency of Feeding

Whether a woman was demand or schedule feeding, many were concerned about the time interval between feedings. Some worried that the baby was feeding too often. Others worried that the baby was not feeding often enough. The following excerpts typify the confusion:

Now I have been actually waking her up and feeding her. I thought I'd better start trying to fatten her up. So I've been trying to feed her more, so that she cries more often for it. I think now that's happening because she's getting more; she's demanding more.

I'm not concerned about feeding too often as long as it doesn't upset her. It always seems that the time I feed her too often is the time she has gas pains. Which comes first, who knows?

The only thing I'm concerned about with feeding too often is that I have read that if you put milk in on milk partially digested, it would all go through and cause more gas because it wasn't properly digested.

In considering the spacing between feedings women thought about themselves as well. Frequent feedings meant that the baby had to accompany the mother wherever she went. Infrequent feedings, in contrast, gave the mother longer rest periods.

Women who were concerned about the length of the feeding intervals usually tried some strategy to change things. They delayed feeds by playing with the baby or giving water or juice. If the baby was sleeping he or she was wakened and fed.

Sara Quandt (1985, 1986), in a study of patterns of breast-feeding behaviour, documented the number and length of breast-feeding episodes per day as well as the intervals between feedings in a group of sixty-two women. At four weeks of age she found that, on average, the babies had seven feedings a day for a total of 141 minutes. The average feeding time was approximately 20 minutes. The average minimum inter-feed interval was two hours and the average maximum inter-feed interval was six hours. The figures at eight weeks of age were similar except that the maximum interval between feedings increased (Quandt 1986). She found that frequent feeding (more commonly associated with demand feeding) correlated with duration of breast feeding. Women who weaned before six months fed less frequently than those who did not wean. Also, mothers who supplemented with formula or solid food fed fewer times per day and fed less frequently (Quandt 1986).

Supper and Evening Feedings

A number of women commented on the frequency of nursing throughout the evening, from supper until bedtime. Many of them voiced frustration over supper-time feedings. They wanted to prepare the evening meal, to have some time with their husbands, and to eat, but found their babies wanted attention at that time, too:

By dinner time my older child is just the pits. The baby at that point wants to be held a lot. Usually I haven't even thought about what I'm going to make for dinner. The dogs are barking and then I get about four phone calls. That's when I'm going 'Aaaagh.'

I know for sure when we have dinner he wants to breast feed even if he's only been fed an hour before. It gets irritating because you want to sit down, relax, have a cup of coffee and a cigarette, and not listen. But you do it anyway.

Women implemented different strategies to cope with the inconvenience of supper-time feedings:

Often I don't eat my dinner until he goes to sleep just because it's easier for me to finish nursing, put him down, and then eat. The nursing is our quiet time so I'm willing to eat later.

Sometimes if he's sleeping and it's getting like 4, 4:30, I just pick him up and feed him because I know if I let him go that at 5, 5:30 he's going to start screaming and that's not a good time for me to be feeding him. I try to work around that time.

It is tough. I do my cooking in the morning, and cook for two days so that by evening I just sit with him and feed him whenever he is hungry.

In some cases the babies were fussy throughout the evening. Comments such as the following were most common around five or six weeks post-partum: 'She has a fussy period in the evening. She just cries and she just wants to be held and bounced and walked and jiggled.' / 'It's such a strange pattern of eating. She'll go on a binge in the evening where she'll eat continuously to make up for lost time. The wakeful time is at night, starting around dinner time and going through. Then quite often she'll go to bed at 11:30 and not want to eat until 7 a.m.'

An evening of nursing or holding the baby, after an already long day, was exhausting and left mothers with even less time for themselves: 'What bothers me is she still has her fussy period starting about six or seven o'clock and goes to nine or ten o'clock. She won't be comforted by my husband. It means that I'm with her, which is a long day.' / 'In the evening she seems to start at six o'clock and go to ten. It just seems that breast feeding has gone on constantly, which is a bit of a drag. I have had no time for myself in the past couple of weeks.'

Some women wondered if their milk supply was down at the end of the day. One woman speculated: 'It seems evening is my bad time. I don't seem to have as much milk but either she has accommodated herself to that or her demands are such that my breast produces the amounts she needs. I still do have less at night, but if I go out and leave a bottle of expressed milk for her, she doesn't take a large amount.'

Other women commented that their babies did not want the breast for nourishment in the evening but instead wanted comfort. Whatever the reason, mothers found prolonged evening feedings time consuming and fatiguing. At best, the time spent feeding in the evening occasionally paid off with a prolonged sleep at night.

Night Feeding

Night feedings were regarded as both precious and a curse: 'The worst part of having a baby is being up in the middle of the night.' The ensuing lack of sleep strained relationships between mother and father as well as between the mother and other children. Even after becoming accustomed to waking in the night, a long feed at that time could be an ordeal. It was one aspect of breast feeding that few women missed when it was over.

No one who spoke about night feeding said it was easy to get up in the middle of the night. Still, there were a number who described positive aspects: 'Once you get up it doesn't bother you really. It's just having to pull yourself out of bed. Once you go in and pick her up it doesn't bother you anymore 'cause she's changing so much. I enjoyed the closeness of her.'

Women with other children cherished night feeds for the privacy and quiet time they had with their babies: 'I used to really enjoy that middle of the night feed. Katharine wasn't there; it would just be Evelyn and I and I wouldn't have to share that time.'

Women also discussed their husbands' lack of assistance with night feedings. Most mothers believed it was their responsibility to handle night feeds, thereby allowing their husbands to sleep and be rested for work: 'Now that he's back at work, he just can't get up at night anymore so it's only me at night.' / 'I really don't think it's fair to wake my husband. I don't mind getting up in the night because I know I can rest during the day.' / 'I'm on leave and my husband isn't. I feel that I should do the night feedings as much as I can because he can't afford to lose the sleep. I can sleep during the day.' Only two women expressed resentment over the fact that their husbands did not have to wake up in the night to feed the baby but they saw no alternative because they had chosen to breast feed.

Night feedings turned into ordeals when the baby did not settle or took a long time at the breast. The frustration and exhaustion that those situations produced is reflected in the following excerpts, both of which occurred when the babies were less than six weeks old.

Breast feeding in the middle of the night is still really the pits. It's one thing when the baby wakes up and cries but then to sit there and breast feed on top of it. I wake up in the night and think, 'I really can't do this much longer.' Every night I wake up in the middle of the night and I think, 'That's it, no more of this.' The morning comes and I forget about it. You're tired enough as it is and nursing makes you even more tired. What keeps me going through that is that soon he'll be sleeping through the night. This is not going to go on forever.

Occasionally a feeding at night would be interminable because of his being very, very restless and having a lot of gas. You feel the gas has been passed, you put him down, and he seems to be quite peaceful. Fifteen minutes later, just as you're drifting off, you hear him crying and nothing seems to soothe him but putting him back to your breast. So a couple of evening feedings have turned into two, two-and-a-half-hour ordeals. Those are times when you really feel very frustrated. You just want somebody else to step in and feed the child or hold him 'cause you're just so tired at that point.

Women persevered despite the exhaustion and frustration of

night feedings because they knew they would not go on forever. Wright, Macleod, and Cooper (1983) found that, on average, babies who are bottle fed reliably sleep through the night two and a half weeks earlier than do breast-fed babies. This takes place at approximately ten weeks of age. The average age at which night feedings stop completely is approximately ten weeks for bottle-fed babies and sixteen weeks for breast-fed babies. The authors concluded that the plausible explanation for this difference was that the breast-feeding mother may be more permissive and therefore less likely to introduce tactics that would encourage the baby to sleep through the night. They found that the longer the mother continued to breast feed, the later the baby stopped feeding at night. This notion is supported by the findings of a study by Cable and Rothenberger (1984) of breast-feeding women who were active members of La Leche League and strongly believed in unrestricted breast feeding. They studied twenty-four mothers whose infants had an average age of seventeen months. They found that 58 per cent of these women were still breast feeding at night approximately 55 per cent of the time. They averaged six suckling episodes nightly. Eighty-eight per cent of the women indicated that the babies slept with them.

Women used a variety of strategies to make night feeding less disruptive or to eliminate it altogether. Some nursed the baby in their beds, particularly in the early weeks following birth. Others described making the night-time feeding as uninteresting as possible so as to not stimulate the baby into complete wakefulness: 'At night I just leave the light out. I nurse her with the light out and change her with a little tiny light. I put her back to bed even though she might be wakeful. In the daytime I try to encourage her to stay awake.'

Some tried, with varying success, to change the baby's feeding time. The mother woke the baby just before her bedtime in an attempt to shift the schedule so she could have more hours of uninterrupted sleep. Some tried to stimulate the baby earlier in the evening, hoping he or she would fall asleep earlier. After a few months most babies began sleeping through the night, but during a growth spurt, night feedings started again. After a period of uninterrupted sleep, the return to wakeful nights was disconcerting. The mothers felt resentful and stressed:

Now that he's getting up in the night he's driving me bananas. Just for the past one and a half to two weeks he's been doing it.

You get used to the night-time feeds. The first month is hard and the second month you've got into a routine and it's fun getting up with the baby – you're enjoying it. Then the baby starts sleeping through except a few times in the night and you're not used to it anymore. I looked at my husband, lying there sleeping, thinking that one night he could get up and give the kid a bottle of milk. I could just sleep for a few hours. I was up every two hours. It's the exhaustion. Your tolerance level drops.

You don't worry about getting up in the middle of the night until you don't have to do it and then you resent going back to it.

Feeding schedules can govern mothers' lives in the first few months. Some mothers want to establish a schedule and their babies are amenable. Others prefer to feed on demand, believing that it is unrealistic for the baby to conform to a schedule. Those who demand fed sometimes faced long evenings with the baby at the breast. Almost all mothers faced feedings during the night and none regretted the passing of that aspect of breast feeding.

CHAPTER EIGHT

Fatigue

Many women found breast feeding exhausting particularly in the early stages. In addition to the physiological stress of lactation there was stress associated with the responsibilities and life-style that accompanied breast feeding. Frequent feedings, long periods with the baby at the breast, night feedings, coupled with the responsibility of caring for other children, the husband, and the house, all contributed to fatigue.

Women talked about how fatigue affected their emotions, their ability to reason, and the physical sensations they experienced. Women mentioned that their patience 'wore very thin' when they were tired. This in turn affected how they coped with everyday activities and events:

My patience is entirely dependent on how much sleep I get the night before. If she has a good night I have the patience of a saint. If she has a bad night, then we're both bad at night and in the day. It gets into a circle 'cause if I'm nervous she picks up on it.

I don't mind the night feedings as long as I can get three to four hours' sleep between them. I have to have my sleep. I can't cope without it. If I didn't get my sleep I would be very afraid because I have no patience. I just wouldn't be able to cope.

The most frequently mentioned consequence of fatigue was arguing with family members. Women recognized they were volatile when tired and knew the arguments resulted from their own fatigue and, in some instances, that of their husbands:

We're not as tired because we're both sleeping through the night. You do tend to take it out on one another when you're tired. We were arguing a lot – over her and anything.

Being up all night, I just really lit into him the other day. I had him upset and me upset. I just realized it was mostly my fault 'cause I hadn't been paying that much attention to him. When you're over-tired your temper is right on the surface.

He's so tired and I'm tired and that's when you're most vulnerable to disagreements and stuff.

Women also described in vivid terms how fatigue affected them physically, especially in the first few weeks at home: 'It's like when I used to work nights and about five o'clock in the morning I'd get feeling sort of nauseated. Sitting in bed feeding him I feel sick. I know I'm not sick. It's this disorientation. There's just no energy, no desire.' / 'If you weren't so tired you could accomplish a lot more instead of dragging around.' One woman described how fatigue resulted in at least one bout of uncontrolled crying: 'My mom left on Saturday. I thought, "This is it now." I was feeling terribly sorry for myself, just crying and crying. I really think it was simply physical exhaustion. It was that type of crying where everything hurts.'

Some women found that the physical and emotional effects of fatigue were not only draining but frustrating. They wanted to do things other than nurse but rarely had the time or energy. When they had the energy, they tried to do too much and merely exhausted themselves again. A lack of a routine was also frustrating but some women felt too tired to set one up. Once the baby began to sleep for longer periods it was easier to establish a routine and their frustration diminished. In some instances, the babies did not settle easily into a routine and the impact was distressing. Lana found she was unable to enjoy her daughter as much as she thought she should because of her fatigue. She was frustrated with her own apathy. At the six-month interview she said: 'She's such a difficult sleeper. I don't enjoy her as much as I would if I were more rested, which is a shame because I know what I'm missing. There's nothing I can do about it. I can't be less tired. From the odd night when I do get a good night's sleep I'm a different person the next day. It's just lovely, but we don't get very many of them.'

One of the difficulties with breast feeding is that the mother is the only one who can do the feeding. A few women found that a bottle of formula or expressed milk, given by someone other than the mother, allowed them a little more sleep. This was not a common solution because so many women were reluctant to interrupt their husband's sleep.

Others were wary of skipping a feeding, kowing that it could interfere with their milk supply. The supply and demand cycle of milk production compounded women's fatigue. When a woman was tired her milk supply was not as good. This, in turn, led to more frequent feedings, which gave the mother less time to rest, which then heightened her fatigue.

Tackling the problem of fatigue must be a top priority in making breast feeding a successful and enjoyable experience. Fatigue amplified emotions, blurred reason, and made coping with isolation and continuous child-care responsibilities more difficult. When there was no relief from these strains women felt tied to their babies and to their homes. These feelings and how they were resolved are discussed in the next chapter.

CHAPTER NINE

Time Commitments

After the birth of a baby time becomes a scarce resource. The demands of a new baby, possibly other children, and household management can easily fill all of one's waking hours, with no time remaining for meeting personal needs. Women reacted differently to these demands on their time. Some were content to devote their time almost solely to baby care. Others found the adjustment more difficult. It took time to come to terms with the magnitude of the responsibilities of motherhood. It was frustrating to be confined to the house. It was depressing never to have time alone to do just exactly what you felt like doing. Breast feeding was a factor in these difficulties because the mother was tied more closely to the baby than she would be if she were bottle feeding. None of the difficulties was insurmountable but they were an important component of the experience of breast feeding.

Feeling Content

Many of the women we interviewed had active, childless lives before the arrival of the baby yet were happy with the life-style changes they had made to adapt to their new circumstances. They gladly limited the time they spent away from their babies so they would be available to nurse. They did not resent living according to their babies' schedules. It helped if they were flexible:

I don't plan anything rigidly. When I have people over for dinner there have been occasions where I missed sitting down to dinner because I'm feeding the baby. It doesn't bother me if he wants to eat in the middle of something. I will stop and feed him or I will wait to go out until he's finished his meal or I plan to feed him where I'm going.

I didn't plan anything. I decided that I'm fitting into her life for the first six months and that's the way it is. That's one of the decisions I had made and there was nothing that I am disappointed with. She's not taking anything away from me.

A number of mothers tried to minimize absences as much as possible. During the early stages, they missed their babies too much to enjoy time away from them: 'I leave him the occasional time. I leave him for an afternoon, two hours. I come back and I can't wait to see him. I miss him so much.' / 'I had a doctor's appointment in the late afternoon. My husband said, "Go shopping, you'd enjoy it." I didn't. I decided I didn't feel like it after all. I don't like being away from him. I miss him so.'

Women recognized the need for some change of scene and chose either to take the baby out with them or to go on short excursions alone.

I enjoyed being with a new-born baby. Sometimes I think the anxiety about getting out is just not worth it. Getting out occasionally and not being totally house-bound makes the difference. I try to get out sometimes during the day and not miss feeds.

Things we're planning – the baby comes with us. I have refused a couple of invitations because I knew that I would be away for an extended period of time. I just wouldn't be comfortable away that length of time. He enjoys being at the breast. It's a tremendous pacifier for him. It's always settled him down whenever he's felt fussy. He gets so excited when he sees me sometimes if I've been away, especially first thing in the morning. His whole body just starts to shake. That's so rewarding.

I've heard a lot of people saying about breast feeding that it ties you down but so far it's not like I really *feel* tied down. My husband wanted to go and see a movie that was very long. I just didn't want to go. I didn't want to leave the baby for all that time. What would I do in the middle of the movie if it was feeding time and there I was in pain and leaking? It just wasn't worth it.

Women who demand fed had to be available at unpredictable times. They worried that their babies would not fare well without them. One mother explained: 'I like to be around if she needs me because when you're nursing you don't know when she wants to feed again. And if I'm not there I feel very guilty.' The baby's comfort was more important to these mothers than their own desire to get out. They were not subordinating their own needs. Instead the baby's needs had become their own.

Feeling Tied Down

Other women we interviewed were less happy with the life changes they had to make. Occasionally they begrudged the lack of time away from the baby or their home. They felt tied down by the demands of baby care and nursing.

About half the women we talked with felt tied down. The term 'tied down' meant different things to different women. There were those who found the continuous responsibility for child care draining. Even if they had time away from the house or the baby, they felt burdened by the responsibility. Others felt tied down simply because they spent a lot of time in the house. They suffered from 'cabin fever' and spoke of being house-bound. When they overcame the obstacles to getting out of the house, they no longer felt as tied down. A third group of women felt tied down because they spent all their time with the baby, yet needed time for themselves. In these cases, an alternate care-giver provided some relief.

Unending Responsibility

There is no escape from the responsibility of child care and this caused some mothers to feel hemmed in or trapped. A mother might get away from home only to discover she still felt restricted because she had the baby in tow. Or she might go out for an evening and discover she did not enjoy it because she knew that she must return to the responsibilities of mothering. Feeling hemmed in arose from knowing freedom was no longer possible yet wanting it anyway. One woman, Rachelle, noted that when she was in low spirits, she wanted to break away from the responsibility: 'I just wanted to leave him and go for a walk but I had to take him with me and that was weird. I couldn't have that feeling of being alone because I wasn't. There are certain times when you feel like there is this growth on you and it's always there and you can't even take a rest.' Rachelle was a single parent and had no one she could rely on to share the responsibilities of child care.

Estelle had a partner but still found that breast feeding was a heavy burden because only she could do it: 'With breast feeding you cannot just say, "Hey, get out of here! Leave me alone for a whole night or a whole afternoon." It's just not an option. Even if there is nothing in particular that you want to do, even if the baby is sleeping well and you feel like you're getting time to yourself, the idea hanging over your head is that you don't have an option.'

Sonja felt tied down because there was no relief from the responsibility for child care: 'At times you feel like a zombie. You just want to get out and get away from it all but you know you're going to have to come back to it anyways. And you feel like you're going to come back to something worse than you left.'

Feeling trapped is a powerful emotion. One woman compared it to having a noose around her neck. It implies that there is no escape. These feelings make it difficult to enjoy fully those rare occasions when the mother finds peace or solitude. Sonja added: 'Like the only time I get to do anything is if we go for a walk to the park or something and he'll fall asleep in the carriage for awhile. But then I still can't do anything.'

Others echoed Sonja's distress. Barb's comments were typical: 'I don't know a thing about time off anymore. It just seems I don't have time off. Even when she's sleeping. It doesn't feel like time off. When my husband is playing with her I know that sooner or later he's going to bring her back to me.' Sometimes guilt could destroy the pleasure of a break, especially if the baby is unhappy: 'When I go out, the baby senses it. He knows I'm not here, and he screams the whole time I'm gone. So when I'm out, I'm feeling really guilty because I know he's screaming. I always make sure I'm home on that three-hour mark for his next feeding. Invariably, every time I come home whoever has been staying with him says, "He's been crying over an hour, waiting for you." It's just horrible. It's really tough.'

The hemmed-in feeling was difficult to dispense with primarily because it focused on the ever-present responsibility for child care and nursing. These responsibilities could never be relinquished for more than a short time.

House-bound

There were a number of women who found it difficult to get away from home, either alone or with the baby. This confinement resulted in a host of feelings and reactions that are captured in the following excerpts:

I'm itching to get out of the house. I'm going to start getting fidgety. I'll want to leave the baby here with the other kids.

It's difficult to explain to people what it's like to have a baby in an apartment and not be able to go out. Claustrophobia, to be locked up in some place. I try not to let it get to me. Sometimes it really depresses you.

You sort of think, 'Well, when am I going to get out of the woodwork?' I feel very disconnected in some ways. The days are just sort of floating by. It's hard to never step outside. It sort of hits you. Wow! I've been in the house for three days in a row. Wouldn't it be nice to walk to the corner. I haven't really had that much opportunity to do that.

Women became restless when they were house-bound. They longed for some stimulation beyond the confines of their homes.
One solution to this problem was to take the baby and get out of the house. There were some obstacles to doing this. A lack of baby transportation was a crucial one. It was essential to have a baby carriage, a stroller, or at least an over-the-shoulder baby carrier. Donna lived in an apartment and her mobility was inhibited because she had no carriage. When the baby was five weeks old, she said: 'I wish sometimes I could pack the two of them together and just go out. It gets so nice outside and here I am stuck inside. The only thing that's holding me back is a pram. If I had a pram I probably would have gone out by now and taken him with me, too.'
Successful use of public transport, such as buses, streetcars, and subways, required that the mother be adept at handling the baby carriage or stroller on stairs and escalators. Lorna, a downtown resident who did not have a car, explained:

I tried taking the baby in the subway. I'm a little uptight about taking the stroller on the escalator. I keep thinking the wheels are going to get caught and I won't be able to get it off in time, so I use stairs. Going down, even though people generally help me, I find very awkward, especially taking her and the stroller and a diaper bag, and getting down the stairs to use the subway. Then I used buses and streetcars, and I've got caught in heavy traffic on a streetcar with the stroller.

Christina, in contrast, found that public transit was a sensible solution to travel needs: 'Ever since my episiotomy healed I have been getting out. Not every day but three or four times a week. I have a stroller for her. I just put her in the stroller and jump on the streetcar. I can pretty well go anywhere.' Women who had cars found it was relatively easy to get out of the house. Those who did not believed life would be much more convenient if they did.

Weather was another important influencing factor. It was difficult to use strollers in snow. Some women were reluctant to take the baby out in the cold, especially a new-born.

The effort required to get out of the house could be a deterrent as well. Sometimes it seemed to be more trouble than it was worth: 'Trying to get out for various medical appointments, things like that. It's always a hassle, getting myself organized, her organized, getting there on time. I have given up ever being on time for anything again in my life.' / 'And then you have to take a big bag with an emergency kit, like diapers and vaseline and wipes and a washcloth, bottle, soother, blanket, and clean sleeper. All those things and that is just for going somewhere for an hour.' This preparation was undertaken grudgingly because it was a prerequisite for getting out of the house. Despite the obstacles, the effort was worth the opportunity to sit in a park, visit friends, or shop because these activities provided a welcome change of pace and a break from the relative isolation of home.

Time for Oneself

As welcome as the excursions from home with the baby might be, they did not allow a mother any time for herself. Baby care and breast feeding, specifically, are extremely time consuming. As one mother said, 'Only you can do it. It really ties you to the baby.' This lack of time without the baby (and other children) was a major reason why women felt tied down.

Mothers wanted time to reaffirm, through adult conversation, that their identity was separate from that of their infants. Some wanted time to do things they had given up when the baby arrived or to get out to do some shopping. Some wanted time to read, sleep, or simply day-dream. When women had gone too long without time for themselves they began to resent the time spent with the baby. Repeatedly they voiced their frustrations:

There were some times that I thought, 'Oh, God why don't I just plug him in and walk around with him.' I really felt quite resentful.

I think that's one of the most discouraging aspects of breast feeding. Feeling that your forays into the real world can only be three hours long because you have to get back in time to feed the baby, and that's a terrible feeling.

I slept over at my dad's. The next day he took care of him while I went shopping. I had to do everything within a certain period of time and ohhh, I felt I was losing my mind.

I'm going out swimming two nights a week. I feed him before I go, but I know I've got to be back. I just can't get in the car and go for a drink somewhere. I have to be back to feed him at 11:30. I just find that too confining. For a little while I was really getting almost angry.

I've had feelings of resentment that I never had any time for myself, that nobody understood that, nobody supported that. I have not had an hour or two to sit and do anything that I want to do for months.

These kinds of feelings were more commonly expressed near the end of the study when the babies were close to six months of age.

The availability of other people to take care of the baby was a prerequisite to time away. In our isolated nuclear families, impromptu help is rarely available:

It's not really anything to do with breast feeding. It's just the baby and having competent people to stay with him while I go out and do something.

It's just that I can't get away from the apartment like I did before. My husband doesn't want me to leave the baby even for a second to go down to do the laundry, so I have to wait for him. He comes home at different times. It's difficult. I feel locked in. No matter how much I want to breast feed, I just want to be able to do my laundry when I want, go out for a walk if I can.

The value of an alternate care-giver was readily apparent when we talked to the women who had one. They were able to enjoy their time away from their children without worry or feelings of guilt. In the examples below family members provided the care-giving services but even then it required advanced planning:

I was out the night before yesterday. I was out for about two hours with some friends. Frank, my husband, baby-sat so that really helped.

It really did us a lot of good to get out on Saturday night. It was our anniversary so we went out for a nice dinner and movie. We didn't rush back. My in-laws came to take care of them. Normally I would have to take the children to them. Then you've got to get the kids out of bed. Going out really does make you feel a little better.

I'm planning my escapes when my mother's here. I'll go get my hair cut and maybe get out shopping or to a movie.

The Importance of a Bottle

If a mother wants more than two or three hours away, then the baby must be willing to take an occasional bottle of either expressed breast milk or formula. This was the key to having some extended personal time. As illustrated in the following excerpts the bottle provided temporary relief from a primary responsibility and allowed the mothers a degree of flexibility and freedom:

I'm already mentally preparing to get lots of milk stored away so I can go Christmas shopping during the day. I can avoid the Saturday and evening shopping. I'll just kind of go off on my own. When I have milk in the fridge I feel quite secure about leaving him.

There were a few times I felt a little bit tied down by the breast feeding. Once I got her to take a bottle I knew if anything did happen, somebody else could feed her. That released me a bit.

Ambivalence

Mothers had to grapple with competing needs. Some made opportunities to get away from the baby only to discover that they felt miserable. Although they wanted to get out and enjoy their social life, they also wanted to be with their babies. For a number of women, leaving the baby even for a short time during the first two to three months led to feelings of regret and sometimes guilt:

It was really nice being out last night. It was the first time without Todd. But part of me didn't want to go. You know, I felt guilty. There was this cute little bundle of joy and I was going out to have a good time. His eyes now are starting to follow me. You do get very protective. What if something happens? I was determined not to call, but I did phone after the movie.

We went to a movie and I had expressed some milk. I was a wreck being away from the baby. Every ten minutes I looked at my watch. I said to my husband, 'This is a really long movie.' It was hard because I'm never away from him.

I always imagine something's going to happen. Nothing ever does happen. She didn't die from hunger. I think she's going to be hungry. I imagine a poor Biafran child.

Ambivalent feelings were common during the months following birth. Familiar patterns were interrupted and life was often in turmoil. Time became a precious commodity.

There was never enough of it to do everything that was important. Women had very little time for themselves. Most of them were tied to the home and some found these restrictions frustrating. Breast feeding was an important aspect of the time commitment, especially during the first three to four months, but it did not necessarily preclude women from getting out or having time away from the baby. However, the availability of trusted baby-sitters and suitable transportation for both mother and baby were important enabling factors. It helped, as well, if mothers were prepared to express breast milk or provide formula if the baby would take a bottle. Even then the outcome was not always uncomplicated. Some mothers had to come to terms with the magnitude of the new responsibilities. Others carved out some free time only to discover that their attention constantly returned to the baby and lessened their pleasure.

CHAPTER TEN

Breast Feeding in Public

The decision to breast feed in public appeared, in large measure, to be based on a woman's perception of its appropriateness and on the opinions or reactions of others when she did it. A decision on where to breast feed is important because it affects the amount of freedom a woman has both outside of the home and in her home when others are present. Of the women interviewed, over half commented on their experiences and feelings about where it was appropriate to breast feed.

Breast Feeding with Family and Friends

The presence of family and friends during nursing generated mixed reactions from the mothers. Most felt comfortable breast feeding in front of female family and friends. A smaller number of women felt comfortable feeding in the presence of male family members and friends as well. Comments such as those below were common:

I did it at parties but most of the people are friends. I'd just sit in the corner and if people happened to see me breast feeding, then it was up to them; they had the choice whether to come where I was, or not.

If my sister comes over and my brother-in-law, and they sit in the family room and it's time for him to eat, I just go on the couch, there in my corner where I always feed him, and feed him.

With my own-age-friends it doesn't matter – men, women, whoever, I just go ahead.

Everyone came around to see the baby; lots of Barry's friends. I wasn't sure how I'd react to that, but it hasn't bothered me at all. She wants to eat and you feed her. I just unzip and unlatch. It's no embarrassment at all.

The cultural heritage of a family influenced the acceptability of breast feeding in front of family members. Two women, whose husbands' families were from different European countries (Scotland and Italy), explained that their relatives were not offended or embarrassed by breast feeding because they were accustomed to it. Two women from other cultural backgrounds believed breast feeding in the presence of men would not be tolerated. They explained that it would be disrespectful or 'they would think I was kind of gross.'

The presence of people of the same generation as women's parents was sometimes inhibiting. Embarrassed fathers, fathers-in-law, and uncles had left the room when some women started nursing. Another woman was asked to leave a restaurant when she started breast feeding because the restaurant catered to older people. One woman compared her reactions to feeding in the presence of a woman of her own age and her mother-in-law: 'If you were with a girlfriend you'd feel quite comfortable breast feeding, whereas if I was with my mother-in-law, she would send me down the hall and close the door behind me because it was just the thing that you didn't do out in public.'

A few women expressed regret over the older generation's views on breast feeding in public but deferred, none the less. Ali's view on the matter was shared by others: 'It's respect for their things. I wouldn't promote something I knew they naturally cannot accept. They're not going to change so I'm not going to embarrass them.'

Some women were surprised to discover that their female friends could not always be relied upon for approval:

Even girlfriends don't like to see it done in public. To me you can't see anything. I have done it fairly discreetly at times.

There were a few women I got into arguments with because they thought it was disgusting.

It's never crossed my mind that there was anything wrong with it. These people's reactions just floored me. All of a sudden here are these sexual connotations to a baby breast feeding. Men and women have said they don't enjoy seeing breast feeding. It's not as though your tits are hanging out. What do they think boobs were made for?

In contrast, women did not expect their male friends to approve of public breast feeding. Repeatedly, they commented that most men regarded breasts as sexual objects rather than a source of nourishment for the baby. 'It might have a great deal to do with women's breasts being displayed as sex objects so that the function as a nurturing vehicle is being played down. When a man sees a woman breast feeding he feels like she's doing something almost obscene. Men may feel it's not discreet to do it in public, that they should do it where nobody sees it.'

The husband of one woman's friend said, 'It's kind of disgusting to see a woman's personal parts.' Some men acted strange in the presence of a nursing woman: 'Grown men turn into little boys. They just act so silly, making such a big deal out of it. Thirty-year-old men act like idiots. It was amazing to watch them all turn into these babbling fools! A couple of them don't have any kids yet. I was getting quite annoyed.'

Women interpreted actions such as these, or prolonged staring, to mean that these men felt uneasy. There were also a few cases where a woman's husband stepped in and discouraged his wife from nursing in the presence of certain friends. These husbands evidently shared the view that public breast feeding was an embarrassment.

Coping with Unease

When people appeared uneasy in the presence of nursing, the mothers reacted in one of three ways. A few remained relaxed and continued breast feeding, believing that the uneasiness of others was not their problem. They were determined not to be deterred from something they believed was acceptable. Sonja explained: 'I say to myself, "Well, you don't want to watch, then you leave the room. This is my corner; this is where I feed him, where I feel most comfortable, and I'm staying here." I do it discreetly.' Another mother said: 'If Beth is hungry and I'm in public, that's tough if it offends their sensibilities. But you can do it discreetly. You can hardly see it.' Fern speculated on people's discomfort: 'I think sometimes people are a little uncomfortable. They don't quite know where to look. They don't know how to react to your enjoyment or the baby's sucking sounds.'

This group of women believed that the sensibilities of others were not their problem, particularly because breast feeding in public could be done discreetly.

A second group of women were uncomfortable nursing in front of others, particularly men, regardless of their reactions. They felt very self-conscious: 'The only negative is my own feelings about breast feeding in front of men. I haven't done it. I've been hiding out. It's a strange and artificial kind of feeling. I've gotten into a routine of closeting myself. It would be a big deal to come out of the closet.' Most of the women who felt embarrassed did not or could not explain why. A few, like Joan, viewed the breast in sexual terms: 'It is a sex symbol. Even myself, when I saw a girl breast feeding on the subway and she was exposed, I felt ill at ease.'

Women who were uncomfortable breast feeding in front of others frequently used the word 'exposed.' They preferred isolation in another room where they were away from prying eyes, embarrassed glances, and the noise and confusion of a large gathering.

The third group of women breast fed in the presence of others when they thought there would be no objection. If the mother was unsure about the reaction she would retire to a private place to breast feed. These women willingly made concessions to avoid embarrassing their friends, in part because the discomfort was infectious: 'There are certain places or situations that didn't bother me at all. If I felt at all that the other person was uncomfortable, then I would feel that, too.'

In an uncertain situation women were usually cautious: 'It's still not really socially acceptable to expose yourself in front of people. No matter how much you say that times have changed they really haven't. You're better off not taking a chance.'

The cost of caution was isolation. Women felt they were missing out on things when they went into another room to breast feed. Their frustration is apparent in the following comments:

I had gone into the dining room to breast feed, although I thought it was stupid having to miss the whole conversation.

The other night we were at a friend's place and Jack was hungry. I had to go into the bedroom and feed him and I was starting to get very aggravated because he eats so much I had to go in there so many times. I had to sit in there for quite a while and I was getting a little bit aggravated that I had to keep going in.

The only pressure about breast feeding is you always have to go somewhere and do it privately. I felt tied down because I had to go away from everybody. It's really stupid.

Breast Feeding with Strangers

Women also talked about nursing in the presence of strangers.

A few would not breast feed in front of anyone they did not know, male or female. They always tried to time their outings around the baby's feeding times. A larger majority of women sought the privacy of washrooms, change rooms, or cars when they needed to nurse.

The few women who chose not to breast feed in the presence of strangers did so for a number of reasons. Pamela mentioned concerns for the quality of the nursing experience for the baby: 'I still think it's private. I still want to be giving him as much attention as possible. I think he notices it, if people are around he doesn't nurse the same way. I think he doesn't feel he's getting his attention because I'm often talking to him.'

Pamela also disliked feeding in front of friends. Her beliefs were probably influenced by her own discomfort as well as her concern for the baby's comfort. Other women expressed views that suggested that nursing in public and exposing one's breast was not proper: 'I'm not all that keen on breast feeding in public anyway. There's contradiction between saying that breast feeding is a very strong connection between mother and child and feeling it's perfectly natural to do it in front of lots of people. I've always felt that there's a certain kind of exhibitionism involved.'

The majority of women said they would breast feed publicly but discreetly. Many talked about certain places being less public than others. Doctors' waiting-rooms or the quiet corner of a restaurant were mentioned as being less public. Women breast fed in those environments, relying on their clothing or a blanket to conceal the breast. Other places were perceived as inappropriate even though the mother was comfortable nursing in public.

I thought about taking the baby with me. I was having lunch at the Ontario Club [a private club], and I didn't see that as the setting to take a baby to. That would have been like feeding the baby in the middle of Creeds [an exclusive store]. It would have been much worse than that in fact, because the Ontario Club is so conservative.

He was screaming for food. So I fed him in the ladies' room in Hazelton Lanes [a collection of expensive shops] and a couple of hours later we were in Holt Renfrew [an exclusive store] and he started to scream again and I ended up feeding him in Holt Renfrew. Those are two places where I said I'll never breast feed a baby, so that was really rough.

Finding appropriate places to nurse was not easy. On two separate occasions Ali had unpleasant and frustrating experiences:

I had a fit at Canada's Wonderland [an amusement park]. They do not have proper nursing facilities and you're not allowed to nurse on the grounds. I went into the lost and found, where I was locked in and the security guard stood outside the door and peeked through every five or ten minutes to see if I had finished yet. I spoke to the supervisor. He said, 'We have a better facility in the hospital section.' So next time around I steered the kids there. We went into the building that was like a hospital and it had nursing mothers. I was behind a curtain listening to women throw up, and a man with back pain so severe he was moaning and crying. It was horrendous.

I was asked to leave Holt Renfrew. I had clothes to try on when she started crying so I sat down and was feeding her. The changing lady came in 'Ah! Oh! Gee!' I said, 'Don't worry it's not a disease, it does not spread. Just give me fifteen minutes.' But she wouldn't go. I fed her and put her down in the stroller. She was screaming and [the clerk] said, 'Maybe you better come back when you can leave your baby at home.'

Violet had a similar experience and ended up having to feed in a particularly open spot:

We thought we could nurse in a changeroom in The Bay. They told us no. We were in The Bay at Fairview [a department store in a mall] in the children's department. We asked, 'Could we nurse in the change room?' She said, 'No, I'm sorry it's not permitted.' We said,

'Where should we go?' She said, 'The main washrooms of the mall are down the way.' That's where we ended up going. There was one chair in the washroom in the combing-your-hair area. We both had to nurse. I was wearing a cape so I went out in the main mall and sat on the bench. He was under the cape. I'm kind of annoyed. I've been downtown at Simpsons [another department store] and nursed in the lingerie change rooms. There's not very much around as far as facilities or at least it's not well known if there is.

Women often had to be resourceful to find a place to nurse:

A couple of times I've been indoors [looking] at the stores along Bayview [a main thoroughfare] and one furniture store there had a quiet little corner back there and the lady running the store said, 'Sure, go and feed her there.' Another little clothing store had a little corner in the back. It was the same thing. So there are ways to manage that kind of thing. Both times it was women running the store and they weren't that busy. If I was in a department store I'd probably just go into a fitting room unless they had their washrooms set up for breast feeding.

It was a chore to have to search out appropriate places: 'I've always found places but still it has become more of a challenge to try to find a place than just being able to go out and know that there is some place where you could go.' Clearly, the lack of facilities was a deterrent to breast feeding in public and was a source of unnecessary problems.

Nursing Facilities: Public Toilets

When women were in public places and wanted a private spot to breast feed they frequently resorted to using public wash-rooms. Often the surroundings were unpleasant and there were no chairs. Women had no choice but to use toilet stalls. They felt strongly about the inappropriateness of wash-rooms as nursing stations: 'It's too bad there are not too many places. Also we don't eat in the wash-room, why should the baby eat in a wash-room? Once she was really crying so I went in the wash-room. I was breast feeding. Every time the poor little thing hears flushing, she would jump in the air. It was terrible.'

As one mother said, 'You have to go inside a wash-room where people void to do something not associated with this.' Another woman who used toilet stalls for privacy and who sat on the toilet to nurse exclaimed, 'How awful, but what else can you do?'

Because privacy was so important many women used public toilets despite the unpleasantness. Even women who did not mind feeding in public would usually prefer to have secluded areas available to them:

I don't care where I breast feed to start off with. I will breast feed wherever it suits me. But if I knew there was a special place that's quiet and away from the crowd I would prefer that. Any woman would.

I used to be incredibly frustrated at the lack of nursing facilities that were available. I was really aware of nursing stations in England. I was really appalled at the complete lack of them here. I think it's important to try to be going out and not be tied down, particularly if you're not used to being at home all the time.

There should be more attention paid to having more facilities. You feel like you're doing something that's not sanctioned.

Government should do something just like they do for handicapped people. It's sort of a handicap because it's something that restricts your freedom of movement.

Women wanted facilities that were private, quiet, clean, comfortable, and separate from toilets. They also suggested that it would be helpful to have a safe play area available for their other children.

Changes in Attitude

Some women's ideas on breast feeding in public changed over

time. In early interviews these women said they would not breast feed in public. They felt embarrassed at the thought of it and thought others would be embarrassed by seeing it. Later their attitudes changed and they began to experiment with feeding in public.

Three weeks after delivery Lana was uneasy breast feeding in public but six months later she was doing it without difficulty. When she first discussed the subject, Lana explained: 'I'm not yet comfortable with feeding her in public because she fusses and I can't seem to do it discreetly. Once I master that I think things will be easier. It's not modesty on my part. I have noticed that some people really find it offensive so I want to be as discreet as possible and make her relax a bit and be relaxed myself. When you are so busy trying to get the areola into her mouth I can't care where my shirt is.'

A week later, Lana was already more comfortable: 'I haven't yet done it in a public place but last night I had a lot of visitors. It was feeding time and I fed her as I was talking to people and there was no problem.'

A month later, Lana went public: 'On Sunday morning we had a brunch and I breast fed her in that restaurant. It was all right. I was able to find a little corner. People weren't really looking at me. It went quite well.'

Little more than three months later, the last of Lana's inhibitions seemed to have disappeared: 'We went to Simpsons [a department store] and I found a couch in front of a restaurant. It was glass enclosed so people could see me sitting on the couch. It was in front of the elevator. That was about the only place I was able to find a spot to sit down and feed her. I put a blanket around her and nursed her there.'

Fiona was surprised to discover that she actually wanted to feed in front of others because it was a public affirmation of a very significant achievement:

There's definitely stages in breast feeding. Right after birth I'm dying to breast feed because I've just read all these books and it's gonna be so wonderful. Then you give birth and it's, 'I hope I can do it.' Then there's infection and all that. The stage then is that I'm comfortable with it. The next thing is where can I feed? Situations have arisen where I said prior to them, I wouldn't feed with such and such people in the room or in that particular circumstance. Then I find that I'm so proud of our feedings that I want everybody to see. I want people to know how I feel proud of myself that I have persevered through all those problems and now here I am breast feeding comfortably. There's this warmth when he feeds that I feel between me and him and I want people to see it.

The shift in attitude toward an acceptance of public breast feeding was not necessarily a permanent one. Despite Fiona's exuberance about nursing in front of others, she noticed that she reacted negatively when a friend breast fed in a restaurant. Fiona was no longer breast feeding at the time:

We were in an Italian restaurant. It came time to nurse and she nursed the baby right there at the table. Even I, as somebody who just finished nursing, was a little bit appalled. I found myself looking around, like is anybody looking? Thinking, 'But Fiona, when you used to nurse in public you used to laugh at people who couldn't accept it.' And now I'm not doing it, I was like – 'This is obscene.' I don't know why I reacted that way. Mind you, I never would have nursed in a restaurant. I just saw it as being completely tactless.

Fiona recognized that her present attitude was a rather dramatic reversal of her recent feelings. Perhaps this demonstrates the strength of attitudes that arise from lengthy socialization. Another woman speculated that in a few years she might marvel at having allowed her breasts to be seen in public. Carol went on to say: 'If you have a baby you lose your modesty for awhile because it's such an overwhelming physical thing. I forget if breast feeding even is supposed to be an immodest thing to do.' Carol noted how the powerful nature of this post-partum time could completely change former inhibitions but recognized that this change might be transient.

The social taboos against public breast feeding have been well documented (Jones and Belsey 1977; Martin 1978). Jelliffe and Jelliffe (1978) noted that the dual roles of women's breasts (sexual on the one hand and nurturing on the other) have led to bizarre situations in the United States where women have been arrested for breast feeding in public. Michele Landsberg reported on numerous instances in Canada where women have been censured for public breast feeding when she was a columnist for the *Toronto Star* and in her book *Women and Children First* (1982).

Deciding where to feed and in front of whom are two of the most controversial aspects of breast feeding. In our industrialized society the breast is still a glorified sexual object and its nurturing functions are of secondary importance in the minds of many. Despite the widespread flaunting of women's breasts that is so apparent in the media, women who breast feed are encouraged to maintain a virgin-like modesty. These inconsistencies guarantee difficulties for breast-feeding mothers unless they manage a studied indifference to their social milieux. Kitzinger (1979) believes that in the face of rapidly changing male and female roles, breast feeding in public symbolizes women coming out of their hidden place, which is threatening to those with traditional viewpoints on women's roles. She contends that women who enter the public arena and breast feed when and where they want are making an important symbolic statement on behalf of all women. This counterbalances the ubiquitous exposure of women's naked bodies in all forms of media, which serves the sole purpose of objectifying women as sex objects.

CHAPTER ELEVEN

The Rewards of Breast Feeding

The rewards of breast feeding centred around the emotional satisfaction of doing something that was good for the baby and around the unique intimacy that developed between mother and baby over the course of breast feeding. The mothers were more likely to emphasize the positive attributes of breast feeding after the baby was a month old and more frequently after the baby reached three months of age. This timing suggests that the more enjoyable aspects do not generally emerge until the baby is two to four months old.

Many women enjoyed breast feeding simply because they found it easy and convenient but the more fundamental satisfaction came from the emotional nurturing and closeness:

I enjoy having my son so close to me, knowing he's getting his greatest pleasure in life from my body, and I'm holding him so close and just watching him sucking and getting his nourishment. He's so close to me and so content. It's just unbelievable.

It's just it's so easy, so comfortable, and the intimacy of the relationship when you're together is so nice. That's why I breast feed.

I felt very womanly and very motherly. With breast feeding I felt very good. It's very hard to know if you've been programmed by reading books and talking to people, and by living in the '80s and being a middle-class person. But I did feel motherly.

For a mother working outside the home the special feelings associated with breast feeding were precious: 'It's that closeness that I would never get otherwise. It's really nice to come home to that.' Other mothers commented that breast feeding enforced a welcome period of relaxation: 'I'll pick her up from her nap to breast feed her and I'll relax and be very comfortable doing it and I think a nice thing about still nursing is that I relax during those feeding times.' / 'It is an escape in some ways, a chance to just sit and relax.'

The mother's belief that she was doing something that was 'right' for her baby was a major source of satisfaction. This was an important factor in the decision to breast feed and often this belief was strengthened by the actual experience: 'We're looking at breast feeding differently now I've actually done it; we're not just looking at it nutritionally. We're looking at it emotionally. We feel that breast feeding had to be the major part of helping him feel secure, content, happy, loved, and nurtured.'

It was gratifying to provide for this unique type of nurturing. The ability to breast feed led to a sense of accomplishment: 'There's a real feeling of pride in being able to do it. I think it's being able to nurture outside the womb. There's a sadness at birth in that the child is gone from me, but to continue nursing, you're keeping that contact.' / 'Nursing a baby successfully really bolsters one's confidence.'

Women discussed the significance of being needed and the singular opportunity of meeting these needs in a way that no one else could. It was a unique part of their lives that was linked to their nurturing, maternal role:

Suddenly when the baby is weaned from you, you're no longer a 'nursing mother.' You're no longer special. You're just one of everybody. Weaning was the giving up of the whole era in my life which has been a very pleasant era. There is something about a pregnant woman or nursing mother that is special.

You are needed. Your child depends on you. It's just a nice feeling – that closeness that you wouldn't necessarily have if it were a bottle and you could just hand the baby to anyone else to feed. It's kind of special.

Persistence

Why is it that some women stop breast feeding, when others, faced with a similar situation, decide to continue? The women we interviewed who stopped early spoke at length about their decision, and their experiences are described in chapters 11 and 12. This section examines why women persisted. There were two critical periods when women had to decide to continue or abandon breast feeding: first, in the initial eight to ten weeks when they were facing the early post-partum strains, and second, when they had breast fed beyond the time they perceived to be the normal stopping time (generally around six months post-partum).

In the early phases of breast feeding, women who found it difficult drew strength from their conviction that 'breast is best.' This was often the only thing that kept them going. The following two excerpts reflect this sentiment: 'I've been home this past month feeding every two hours during the day and three hours at night, and I'm thinking, "When is it going to stop?" It's because I know I'm doing the right thing, and that I want to do it, that keeps me going.' / 'I just want so much what's right for her. That just is too strong a desire for anything else to be significant.'

Another source of will-power was a faith that the difficulties would pass. Those who had breast fed before knew from experience that things would improve. First-time mothers had to rely on their own belief or assurances from books or friends. It helped to take one day at a time. A new day might bring a change or, at least, some respite:

Everyday I think, 'How much longer can this go on?' Actually it's just during the night that I think that way 'cause I'm so tired. I wake up in the morning and I'm fine again. I think, 'Well, certainly, I'm not going to stop.'

My nipple was so sore and I was ready to give up. I kept thinking, 'Well, it's almost over.' They'll be toughening up soon and each day I noticed they weren't quite as painful as the day before. I persevered and I was determined. I just kept thinking of all the work involved and having to do bottles and I thought, 'No, I won't bother.'

It also helped if the mother had been prepared mentally for potential difficulties. The following examples illustrate how such an awareness helped mothers accept breast feeding as a process that takes time to establish comfortably: 'I think I'm going through an initial difficult time right now, but I realize it's not going to last forever and I realize it's very common.' / 'I would think breast feeding is something you have to work at. I anticipated that beforehand. I'm not too upset that I don't find every time I sit down, it's the most wonderful experience in the world, 'cause we still have to work things out.'

For a few women, commitment to finishing a task that was started was important, particularly when they had struggled so hard to succeed: 'My husband thinks I should think more of myself. He thinks I should try and switch to the bottle because he thinks it's just been too hard on me. I really can't. It seems like such a crazy thing to do at this point in time when you're verging on getting her settled and everything is settling out a bit better.' / 'I really struggled a lot to get the ease of where it is now. He's doing well, he's healthy, he's thriving on it. It's a reason to continue.'

For many women, simply continuing was an important factor in perseverance because the longer they breast fed the more opportunity they had to experience, first hand, some of the enjoyable aspects that were described earlier in this chapter. It underscored the unique closeness they felt while breast feeding and the soothing effect nursing had on their babies.

Once women moved beyond the more difficult early months the question shifted from whether they might *stop* breast feeding immediately to how long they would *continue* breast feeding. Once the six-month point was reached a number of mothers commented on why they were persisting beyond that time period. It seemed as if they felt some necessity to justify why they were not stopping, whereas earlier they were emphasizing the perseverance that was necessary to continue.

Almost three-quarters of our mothers were still breast feeding at six months, and 42 per cent of the group we followed to one year were still breast feeding at that point. By six months the majority of women enjoyed breast feeding and found it very easy to do. Many believed that bottle feeding would be far less convenient and a few expressed an antipathy to formula. Some women wanted to prolong breast feeding because they planned no more children and so cherished the few remaining weeks and months. Other women, particularly those who were not working outside their homes, stated that they could simply see no reason for stopping.

The majority of women did not want to wean until the baby appeared ready. Some had assumed the baby would be ready at a predetermined time but postponed weaning when it was apparent that this was not the case: 'After about four months I said, "I'll start gradually to wean until six months." But she didn't want the bottle so now I'm still breast feeding.' / 'I definitely knew I was going to breast feed until he was six months old, then I'd see after that how he behaved. Obviously he doesn't want to be weaned. I can tell what's going to calm him down. If he starts getting upset, I will just plug him in. That's fine. It doesn't bother me if I do it 'til he's eleven months.'

Women had other reasons for postponing weaning. A few disliked the thought of a bottle and held off weaning until the baby could go directly to a cup. This comment was typical: 'I don't want to get him onto a bottle. I'd like him to go straight from drinking at the breast to a cup. I hate to see kids walking around with bottles hanging out of their mouths or the idea of them going to bed and lying in bed with it half in their mouths and rotting their teeth.'

Others were reluctant to wean because they cherished breast feeding. They toyed with stopping but could not bring themselves to do it. The following excerpts capture their sentiments:

I was going to wean him this month then I just couldn't bring myself to do it. I feel like I'd be losing my baby when I wean him. When I tried a bottle it was really a shock. It was just as if I'd lost a little bit of him already. It's that feeling of his losing his dependence on me. Having someone need you is a very good feeling. I know he'll always need me for one thing or another but weaning him will just be one tie that I've broken.

I'm not looking forward to giving up breast feeding because it's letting go of my baby. It's a hard thing to explain – giving it up would be a sign like she's growing up. It's just something we do together and I don't want to give that up.

Breast feeding is a very profound experience for both mother and child. I get really upset sometimes, when I consider giving it up, because I know that I'll never be as close to her again. And she'll never be as close to me again. It's sort of like the empty-nest syndrome you go through later, when your children leave you. They no longer need you anymore.

The beginning of weaning was often the trigger to decide to breast feed longer. Once mothers began the process they decided they did not want to stop and so continued with both breast and bottle feedings: 'I found it really hard to give him a bottle and feel he was getting anything good. I almost feel I was giving him junk food. I still find it hard. I couldn't take him right off the breast now. I don't know how long I'm going to feed him. I'm going to have to stop some day.' / 'It's been over two months that he's getting two feedings from the breast. I like it because I feel it settles him down at night especially. When he wakes in the morning I don't have to be bothered with heating the bottle and all that.'

A few women persisted because of the perceived benefits to the baby. Although their personal enjoyment was less pronounced than that of other women, they continued to breast feed. The following excerpt illustrates the mixed emotions that are involved:

I've had such a rough time with her and with breast feeding that I haven't always felt that it's as wonderful as people make it out to be. More of it was an intellectual thing rather than an emotional thing with me. My emotions were such that, at times, I wish I hadn't. I wouldn't have had to go through so much. On the other hand, I guess we have to measure it off with the fact that she is doing well regardless and seems to enjoy it. It is so easy. I do enjoy it but I persevere more for the intellectual reasons like knowing that it's good for her and preferring it for her 'cause it really hasn't been a piece of cake for me. But I'd still breast feed the next one, for those intellectual reasons.

Two other mothers who breast fed for six months commented: 'It is fabulous for the baby. That's why I'm doing it. In terms of fabulous for the mom – I can't vouch for that. I certainly don't see stars and the earth doesn't move.' / 'I'm not wildly ecstatic about it, the way you read about in books when they say it's such a moving experience. I don't find it particularly exciting.'

These comments imply that some women are led to believe that they would find breast feeding extraordinarily gratifying. Such expectations need to be tempered because, as is evident elsewhere in this book, the mismatch between expectations and reality can be a factor in early weaning. From the examples cited above, mothers might be reassured to know that not all women are delighted by breast feeding yet carry on with it quite successfully.

The question of why women persist in breast feeding is a difficult one to answer in a tangible way. Sheer determination appears to be the single most important factor. Determination arises from a strong belief in the value of breast feeding and from an optimistic spirit. It is reinforced when mothers experience the benefits. In fact, as the benefits became more obvious, many of our mothers were reluctant to stop unless there was a compelling reason to do so.

A Case Study

One of our mothers, Fern, spoke eloquently about the very deep satisfaction she derived from breast feeding. To complete this chapter, Fern's experience is presented in detail because her comments capture the essence of the positive elements of breast feeding.

Fern was thirty-four and expecting her second child when we began interviewing her. Her first child, a boy, was two years old. She had breast fed him for seven months. Fern's attitude toward breast feeding had changed during her first pregnancy: 'Breast feeding was something that was very foreign to me. My mother never breast fed any of her four children and I was never around anyone who breast fed. I remember being repulsed by it. I remember before I was even married thinking, "Oh gosh, I could never do something like that." I guess I thought you had to be more comfortable with your own body.'

The reading Fern did during this first pregnancy convinced her that feeding would be the easiest, best, and most natural way to feed her baby. She recalled her experience of breast feeding her first child for seven months: 'It was just such a positive experience. The most positive part was the bonding that I felt with my child. I mean here I was nurturing him and it was just the two of us and no one could come in on that experience. So I enjoyed it very much. I felt a little lost when I stopped the first time. It was the last link, exclusively, between me and my baby that I was giving up.'

Fern was hoping to breast feed her new baby even longer. Having learned from her first experience, she was hoping she would be more flexible this time, particularly about schedules:

I'm probably a little wiser this time. The first time I was trying to fit everything more into a schedule. There were times when Donald was fretful but I didn't offer him the breast because maybe I had fed him half an hour before. But on talking to some other people and watching a friend whose breasts seemed to be constantly in her baby's mouth it seemed to work. The baby was obviously quiet and enjoying himself. So I think this time I might be a little more flexible in my attitudes towards it and not try to put the baby in a perfect little schedule that would fit me rather than the baby.

The birth of Fern's second baby was traumatic. The cord was flushed out when Fern's water broke and the baby's heartbeat was lost. An emergency Caesarian was then performed and the baby was born within four minutes of the waters breaking. In the months that followed, Fern found it difficult to get over the trauma of nearly losing her baby. During her six-month interview she spoke of how depressed she had felt during the first month post-partum and of her compelling need to talk. (Fern noted how valuable it was to talk to the interviewer who was the 'one person that I could just pour my heart out to.')

In addition to this trauma Fern encountered many of the same difficulties that are described earlier in this book. She had severe nipple pain in the first three weeks and her breasts leaked profusely for the first few months. She was exhausted during the first six weeks and described herself as weepy and sensitive. Her fatigue was compounded by her slow recovery from the Caesarian section. One month after the delivery Fern felt depressed because of being overweight and she wanted to lose 20 pounds. Her two-year-old resented the baby at times. Her husband was having difficulties at work and was consumed with making a decision about whether or not to seek alternative employment.

Despite these factors Fern was delighted with breast feeding. Learning from her first experience she was determined to relax and enjoy the period of infancy. To convey the character of successful breast feeding a series of excerpts from the interviews with Fern are presented. In these passages Fern not only described what it was she found so enjoyable but also commented on attitudes that helped make her experience more rewarding.

In the second post-partum interview Fern was coping with tender, painful nipples. She knew from breast feeding the first child that this would pass: 'It's just an emotionally satisfying experience. Physically it's not that uncomfortable that I would ever consider stopping. The benefits far outweigh the thirty seconds of discomfort that I might feel at the beginning. And I think that it will get better as my nipples toughen up a bit as well. I know some women have a lot of pleasant feelings but I can't say physically that I do. It's more an emotional thing for me.'

At three weeks post-partum Fern was noticing a difference in her response to the new baby. She recalled that, with her first child, things had to be 'just so.' She remembered 'ranting and raving' if things were not 'just so perfect that you could snap a picture and say isn't this lovely.' She elaborated: 'I spent most of my breast-feeding experience reading at the same time, usually child-care books, and I was just right up on everything Donald should be doing and how I should be responding. I'm not into that this time at all. None of that stuff really matters. It's just the love that's there when you're with your child. I'm just sort of more relaxed. I can just sit back and enjoy my infant more.'

As a result of these attitudes Fern found breast feeding relaxing. At times it even allowed her the opportunity to escape from other responsibilities:

I find when I am breast feeding and my mind is totally a blank that it's good in some ways but other times I'll look down at this baby and think, 'Well, I should be talking to you or cooing or something' but then I'll just throw my head back and sit there. I don't know whether it's just the fatigue but I remember relating more verbally with my first than this one. I'm really not sure whether it's a good or bad thing but there have been occasions when I'm just a lump and very relaxed. I'll come to every once in a while and talk to him and then just drift off into nothingness again. So it certainly is relaxing.

Fern's shift in attitude towards demand feeding meant that the second baby was put on the breast whenever he cried excessively or was particularly fussy. She found this approach, ultimately, to be 'far less taxing' than feeding on a schedule and 'pacing all evening long with a screaming child,' which is what she did with her first-born. Fern found demand feeding to be a solution to fussiness and despite the time demands she drew considerable satisfaction from her ability to soothe the baby through breast feeding:

This past week there's been two occasions where single women have been visiting and I just seem to have had the breast out all the time. They're a little taken aback, saying, 'You just sit there and feed this child all the time.' And my sister was here on one occasion and he was really fussy at meal time so I just fed him at the table. She said, 'You've been feeding that child for about four hours straight.' And I said, 'Well, he seems happy and content.' But I think it may have put her off a little bit. I tried to explain to them that it's good for both of us. I find it satisfying for me and it's certainly benefiting Samuel because he's putting on weight and is healthy so it's just a period of time in both our lives.

For Fern, the trade-off for the time on the breast was a messy house and casual meals but the satisfaction from breast feeding made it an acceptable compromise:

The house is an absolute shambles. The dust is an inch thick. The other day I took my two breast pads, which were a little damp, and dusted the stereo with them because I looked down and thought, 'Oh my gosh, this is so embarrassing,' but the place is an absolute mess. My husband picked things up on a couple of occasions but I don't even bother; I just sort of step over things and move things aside. I just manage to get the garbage out twice a week and that's it. I get a good meal on the table at dinner time occasionally and the other times it's grilled cheese and soup but we're all surviving. We seem to be coping far better this time than the first time.

Breast feeding had a tranquilizing effect on Fern. While coping with two children and the aftermath of a traumatic birth, Fern was also trying to be supportive of her husband as he grappled with his employment-related problems. In the face of these difficulties breast feeding provided a welcome respite: 'The few times that I have been really upset I find that the one thing that will relax me is sitting down and breast feeding Samuel. Because I find everything else leaves my mind at that time and I'm just relating to him and enjoying him and sitting back and relaxing. So that's been one life-saver for me – the breast feeding.'

Fern made other comments about the personal importance of breast feeding. When asked how she would feel if she had to stop, she replied: 'Very upset. Very upset. It would be like cutting the ribbon. There's this bond. There's the two of us that are a unit. We're one at this point in time while I'm feeding and I would miss that terribly.' In the same interview she said: 'Breast feeding is a joy for me, an absolute joy – I love every minute of it.'

The baby's development led to more interaction between Fern and her baby and breast feeding enhanced the interaction:

In the past few weeks I've sensed a change in that he is not as demanding of the breast as he used to be. So we can sit back and look at one another and smile at one another and play all those little games and that's enjoyable. Whereas at the beginning I enjoyed it and even though he was always at the breast we didn't have the time for the interaction or he wasn't old enough to interact. But now his face lights up when he sees me smile at him. So I guess that with the two together it's certainly very pleasurable.

Previous experience with breast feeding helped Fern enjoy it more the second time around. She was not as overwhelmed by so many new things and was able to focus more on the enjoyable aspects: 'There were just so many things that I was being bombarded with, with the first child, that I couldn't really isolate the breast feeding experience for what it was. All those other things still go on but I just feel I'm taking more time with the breast feeding and thinking about it more and enjoying it more.'

It is obvious from Fern's comments that, rather than viewing breast feeding as a burden, she saw it as a privilege. Although her first experience had been positive, Fern had learned what approaches could enhance her enjoyment so that the second time she could fully enjoy it. Many women might envy her, for, as she noted in the following quotation, breast feeding can be a unique and rewarding experience: 'I find there's a bond between women who have breast fed. If you're visiting someone and the occasion arises to feed your child you can just see their eyes light up and they start to reminisce about their own experiences and how much they did enjoy them and miss them, too. You know, that's one part of mothering that's so pleasurable and I think those feelings stay with you for a long time, probably forever.'

Numerous books have been written about breast feeding. They discuss why it is appropriate, the technical aspects of breast feeding, and approaches to solving the various problems that might emerge over the course of breast feeding. Because so little emphasis has been placed on understanding breast feeding from the mother's point of view and through her own choice of words, there are very few accounts of the actual meaning of breast feeding and, indeed, of the meaning of nurturing children. Although there is a strong, informal culture that exists among women that supports breast feeding, its meaning for women remains largely unarticulated. Michele Landsberg noted this gap in her book *Women and Children First* (1982:166):

Between these two moments, the early nurturing and the weaning, lay ... a time of enfolding intensity that I have never known in any other kind of love or work. I'm quite sure that this mother time was the making of me as a person, and the making of my three children. Yet I've never seen this fundamentally important interaction recognized or ever acknowledged in films, newspapers, magazines, television, popular music, or any of the aggressive, tawdry, or sentimental noise that passes for our culture, and even to speak of it is to put oneself in a defensive and somehow ludicrous minority. This worries me.

Dorothy Smith, a feminist sociologist, would argue that this absence of women's voices on topics that are vital to their lives is no accident. In her book, *The Everyday World as Problematic: A Feminist Sociology* (1987), she describes how issues and concerns that arise out of women's experiences have never become an important part of the broader intellectual and cultural world that becomes established through the written word. She stresses the importance of shifting our attention to the nature and expression of women's experiences and to comprehending the social processes that influence it. She notes, however, that because we have little experience in speaking of our lives it is hard to find the words to express what is happening to us. In some respects the data from this study support her contention. The women we interviewed were able to discuss the day-to-day problems and concerns about breast feeding but it was more difficult to articulate the essence of what the experience as a whole meant to them. So when the time came to write a chapter on the more abstract aspect of the rewards of breast feeding the data were not as rich. This is not because there were no rewards; these women breast fed for longer than most Canadian women and were obviously highly committed to it. It is more likely, as Smith suggests, that we lack the images, concepts, and frameworks to express the distinctive and significant aspects of our experiences. Among the women we interviewed Fern was a notable exception. She was able to capture and express her feelings and thoughts about the unique role of breast feeding as a means of nurturing children.

PART FOUR

Weaning

The Canadian Paediatric Society (1979) recommends that breast milk is the best source of food for the first six months of life. The figures presented in chapter 2 indicated that although Canadian women are still some distance from reaching that goal they are moving in the right direction. Ten to fifteen years ago well over half of Canadian women who breast fed had stopped within three months. Upwards of 30 per cent had stopped within the first six weeks – before lactation was fully established. Since that time these figures have changed dramatically. The number of women stopping within the first six to eight weeks has been cut in half. The number of women still breast feeding at three and six months has doubled (McNally et al. 1985; Tanaka, Yeung, and Anderson 1987).

The women in our study breast fed much longer than most Canadian women. At four months only 16 per cent had stopped breast feeding and at six months only 26 per cent had stopped. This compares with Ontario averages from the Ross Surveys (Ross Laboratories, personal communication, 31 January 1989), which found that at four months 58 per cent of women had stopped breast feeding and at six months 74 per cent had stopped. Clearly the women in our study were highly committed to breast feeding.

The experiences of women who weaned within the first four months of breast feeding are presented in chapters 12 and 13. Weaning is defined as the point at which the baby no longer received any breast milk. Babies who were weaned prior to four months were considered to have been weaned prematurely. Four months was selected because it is the minimum time period of the standard maternity-leave benefits. It also seems to be a psychological marker as many of the women who stopped prior to four months believed they were stopping 'too soon.' Obviously, factors other than this belief played a major role in determining the timing of weaning. Women's experience is presented in detail in the hope that these accounts will help others avoid the pitfalls faced by these mothers, particularly those whose experience was traumatic. The experiences of those who weaned between four months and one year are presented in chapter 14.

CHAPTER TWELVE

The Decision to Wean Early

Most mothers who stopped breast feeding prior to four months responded in one of two ways. One group of women experienced considerable distress as they grappled with a decision to introduce a formula supplement and then wean. For the second group of women the decision was a straightforward one and was accompanied by minimal distress. In many instances the reasons for weaning were similar in both groups. It was the mother's emotional response to making the decision that was characteristically different.

Distressed Weaning

Over half the women who stopped breast feeding prior to four months found weaning distressing. There were a number of markers that signalled the distress. These included a sense of deep disappointment, frustration, uncertainty, doubt, and feelings of inadequacy and guilt.

Women's expectations about what breast feeding would be like represented an important factor. When expectations were not met the disappointment was profound. In many instances women were unable to be explicit about their expectations ahead of time. However, in face of the daily reality of breast feeding they discovered that they had anticipated something quite different.

The following series of quotations from Jane, a first-time mother whose difficulties with breast feeding began from birth, illustrate the interplay between her expectations and her actual experiences: 'At this point I can't see the light at the end of the tunnel. I had thought it's just going to be a wonderful feeling having this baby at your breast and touching, and it hasn't really been that. The only wonderful feeling is when he's not feeding and I've got him lying on me.'

Two weeks later Jane spoke at length about what she had expected of herself and of how she was slowly coming to terms with these expectations:

I think I was somewhat unrealistic about the whole thing of how much work a baby is. I'm just not used to putting aside everything else and then being tired too. I've got to realize that it is OK for me to be fast asleep when my husband comes home at 6, and I don't have to apologize for it and it's OK after two o'clock in the afternoon to just crawl back into bed and go to sleep for two hours if you've been up at night. But your mind tells you no, you've got to go make a souffle, or you've got to do whatever. I found it difficult to accept that not everything is 100 per cent perfect. Perfect meaning having a good baby and a good marriage and nice house and good breast feeding going 100 per cent OK, and doing all the quote 'right things' in *Better Homes and Gardens*.

If a woman's expectations were exceptionally unrealistic it added insult to injury because she felt foolish for having been so naïve. Betty, one of our first-time mothers, is a case in point. In the pre-birth interview she expressed optimism about breast feeding, believing it would unfold naturally. She viewed it romantically: 'I'm a great believer in letting nature take its course. I think you can make yourself anxious and get yourself worked up over something that should come naturally and be very relaxed. Everything going perfectly – that's the way I picture breast feeding. That's the epitome of breast feeding. That would be what it's all about.'

In actual fact, breast feeding turned out to be very difficult and Betty felt silly: 'I thought it was just me that had this fairy-tale idea. I feel really stupid – admitting to people all these ideas that I had about childbirth and babies and breast feeding. They're fairy tales. I find it ridiculous that I could be 32 years old and still have this naïve idea. It's kind of embarrassing to think that you could be that naïve about something that happens so repeatedly. It just absolutely flabbergasted me.'

Both Betty and Jane wished they had been better prepared for what to expect and wondered why they had not read or heard about some of the difficulties they encountered. They both described being prepared for only minor difficulties and felt isolated and unique when they ran into problems. They discovered later that others had faced similar problems but had not shared them: 'I had girlfriends say that their husbands had been really concerned that they were ready for the loony bin. Another girlfriend had problems with breast feeding; I find out all this afterwards. Before nobody mentioned it. I guess it's not something that they really want to spread around – like "I was a mental case."'

Mercer (1981) has labelled this process of reconciling expectations with reality 'grief work.' It is one of the foremost concerns of some women in the early post-birth period. She noted, as well, that during this time women experienced a period of heightened vulnerability and were highly critical of themselves. In another article Marut and Mercer (1979) noted that women felt ashamed of their self-perceived 'failures' and worried that others would view them as weak.

Much of the disappointment expressed by the mothers centred around their inability to do something they believed in so strongly. As noted earlier, almost all the women in the study were keenly aware of the positive benefits of breast feeding and valued it highly. One mother, Mary, expressed her disappointment poignantly a number of times in her six-month interview. Having successfully breast fed her daughter nine years earlier, she described her view of breast feeding: 'I think that contact from breast feeding is really

really necessary. If you don't have that I think there's something lacking. It's not maybe 100 per cent, it's only 75 per cent. If you went with the breast feeding you're getting that extra 25 per cent.'

Mary's second child was colicky and neither breast feeding nor anything else soothed the child. Mary was at a loss to know what to do. In desperation, she was willing to try anything and switching to formula seemed a viable alternative. Because she believed so strongly in breast feeding, Mary felt torn. She spoke about what breast feeding meant to her: 'It's very emotional. It's like love. I mean how can you explain love? How do you put it into words? It's beyond explaining. It's a definite bond – a closeness. It's the same thing but on a different kind of level than when you fall in love. Everything is rosy and all that sort of stuff; an "in love" feeling. Of course, you don't have the same sexual thing. But there's the same sort of one on oneness – a specialness.'

Given her strong beliefs Mary was saddened by her decision to wean. She believed she and her son were missing something important. She felt like a failure:

So I had feelings of failing because of the C-section and I had this thing with the breast feeding not working. That's part of the reason why I didn't want to finish breast feeding. It was finishing on such a negative note. I wanted it to go good before I finished. Then I wouldn't look back on it as being a negative experience. I didn't want that. Carol was such a positive experience. I wanted to establish the same rapport with Tom as I did with Carol. And I never felt that I got the chance. I felt breast feeding was part of getting that rapport. In some ways I felt that was why I was having these negative feelings towards Tom. All that surge of love just wasn't there.

In almost all the distressing incidents of early weaning the baby was unhappy. She or he was fussy, gassy, cried excessively, wanted frequent feedings, and had long periods of sleeplessness. In some instances these symptoms were described as colic. Whatever they were labelled, they had a marked impact on the mother. Many simply did not know what to do and felt helpless and desperate. The following excerpt from an interview with Betty illustrates these feelings:

It's just another whole dimension of feelings. You can't imagine how deep they go. You just feel you can't do enough. When things start going wrong it's just devastating. You can't see the end of the tunnel. You don't know how long you're going to have to cope like this – if it's just a temporary state or if it is going to last for a long time. It was a real big adjustment. When they start crying you think you've done everything possible, and you've fed them and watered them and in your mind there is absolutely no reason for the crying. Then you get really upset thinking is there something wrong with her or what have I done? I'm sure that the tension with all this being new and no sleep and trying so hard and not knowing what you're doing is definitely there. Everything is overwhelming – the responsibility and the lack of knowledge and the coping in general is unbelievable. I looked at a couple of teenagers and I thought, gee, there they go, not a care in the world. I'm feeling that a lot.

Another powerful feeling accompanying weaning was a sense of inadequacy. Some mothers believed they must be incompetent because breast feeding was not going well or because their child was unhappy. Jane alluded to these feelings as she described an event that was very upsetting to her. Her son was hungry but was fighting the breast and refusing to suck. He arched his back and screamed. Jane, in an attempt to calm him, changed his diaper, which only aggravated his behaviour. Her husband then came in and took over. Jane described her feelings about this incident: 'I felt really bad. Like why does he have to come to my rescue? Why can't I do this? Why does he have to take over? You could see that Mark and I were just at odds with each other.'

Eleanor had introduced formula within two weeks of birth because she was concerned that her milk was slow to come in and felt her baby was not getting enough to eat. On numerous occasions she linked her ability to breast feed to her competence as a mother. She described these feelings in retrospect: 'I had a real crisis of confidence at the beginning. It was clear that she was not taking to it well. I felt if I can't breast feed my baby there's something really wrong with me.' Betty, too, recalled such feelings: 'I remember feeling so inadequate as a mother because I was having so much trouble that I couldn't satisfy her. It's so easy to think I'm not doing anything right.'

Because of their strong convictions about the value of breast feeding many women battled guilt as they tried to decide whether they should wean. Jane struggled with her guilt but concluded she had to switch to formula: 'I felt very very guilty on the weekend that I'm giving it up. But over the last few days I have been fine. This is my decision and I am entitled to do what I know is right.' Betty felt similarly: 'I felt so guilty. I was sort of between a rock and a hard place. You feel damned if you do, damned if you don't. For me the supplement was just fantastic. I know that the baby does fine on formula – I didn't know that then. And I do better as well.'

The term 'failure' was used repeatedly by these women. These feelings were particularly strong for both Jennifer and Laurie. In both cases their physician had suggested that they supplement breast feeding with formula at the end of a feeding because of concern about insufficient weight gain. Both mothers had strong reactions that included feelings of confusion, anxiety, and guilt. Both were sceptical about their physicians' view of adequate weight gain and were uncertain about what to do. Laurie eventually changed doctors but the seeds of doubt had been planted and both women introduced formula. Although Jennifer did not switch physicians she lost confidence in her doctor and later concluded that she would not have weaned when she did if he had not suggested supplementation.

The was only one woman in the group who found weaning distressing whose situation was significantly different from those described above. Kim was unhappy breast feeding her baby. Her older child was jealous and difficult. Kim wanted more of a routine, more free time, and help with the feedings.

She quickly came to the conclusion that breast feeding was not right for her but she persevered for five weeks because her husband wanted her to. She and her husband were in conflict during this period and Kim was frustrated, angry, and unhappy until she stopped breast feeding.

Women's reactions after weaning varied. For some, it was a satisfactory resolution and mothers felt comfortable and even happy with the outcome. After weaning Jane said: 'I'm glad I tried breast feeding. I'm glad I had enough sense to stop. I really am, because the relationship would have just started to go downhill with the baby and with my husband.' She also reflected on what she would say to other women who are experiencing problems: 'My advice to people who were having trouble is to really take a good look at all the areas: how they feel about it personally, and how their relationship is with their baby, and whether that's being compromised because of the difficulties that they are having with breast feeding. Because you can be doing more damage than you are doing good.'

Betty weaned more slowly than Jane and thoroughly enjoyed the eight-week period when she fed both breast milk and formula: 'I cannot tell you the pressure that went off my head when I had that bottle. It was like, "I can breathe again." Because I felt such responsibility for having to be up every time she wanted to be fed, and not being able to leave for five minutes to have my own space. It was just a tremendous relief. When I did want to breast feed I enjoyed it so much more because the pressure wasn't there. It is a tremendous responsibility.'

Some women, while not delighted with the outcome of weaning, accepted the situation with equanimity. For example, Julie had to stop breast feeding after three and a half weeks because her baby would not suck. Before introducing formula Julie tried three days of constant breast feeding accompanied by rest and fluids for herself. She felt certain that she had done all she possibly could and was therefore at ease with her decision.

At the other end of the spectrum are Eleanor, Jennifer, and Mary, who all felt regret and sadness over the way things worked out. Some of the regret came from second-guessing the decision to use formula in the first place. In the following quotations from her six-month interview Mary recalled her disappointment and ambivalence:

I was sorry afterwards that I finished because I didn't want to stop. When I started to wean I still had this feeling that I kept wanting to do it. My husband kept saying, 'Haven't you weaned him yet?' I kept saying, 'No, I have to feed him one more time.' I didn't want to let go. It was like cutting off a bond, a very sort of special bond. I really didn't want to do it. This is more at the emotional level than at the physical level. I mean I didn't want to let that go. I really didn't. And even now I still regret it.

In some ways I felt that my husband was forcing me into it. You have two forces at play – logic and emotion. My husband was very logical about the whole thing. And you could quite understand that because he was not as emotionally involved as I. To my husband it's a source of food and that's it. The source of food wasn't working out and the baby was not happy and therefore was changed to a different source of food. It was just very straightforward. Very, very logical. With me it was a lot more emotional. It was like the Caesarian section. It was a disappointment. I stopped breast feeding to see if we could settle Tom down. But I didn't want to take such a drastic step in settling him down. If the bottle wasn't going to help, if he was a colicky baby, well then, I've given up breast feeding for nothing. It's a real emotional state. At that time I really did not feel capable of making decisions. I felt I couldn't logically look at things and say I should do this or I should do that.

Comfortable Weaning

The second group of women who weaned early were those who arrived at their decision with relative ease. Each one of these women had been clear about her intentions in the pre-birth interview. Each intended to breast feed either for a specific period of time (because of returning to work or simply because that was the length of time that was acceptable to them) or only until problems arose that seemed unmanageable. The following excerpts from the pre-birth interviews illustrate these intentions:

If breast feeding is not going to work then I'm not going to fight nearly as hard as I did the last time because I've got another child to think about. It's not that I want to admit failure but I do want to feel that I'm going to be a lot more sensible because I really fought far too hard the last time and perhaps that was detrimental in itself.

I intend to breast feed but I don't know for how long. I have no plan and no desire to progress to a particular length of time. How long I go on will just depend on how easily it all fits in. If it became a trial and tension, I probably won't do it.

I'm going to play it by ear. I'm going to see how it works and if I'm too tired then or if it just doesn't pan out, I'm not going to commit myself to that. I'm not so idealistic about it that I'm going to commit myself to something that is too hard on me.

Each woman in this group eventually decided to add supplement and to wean prior to four months post-partum. The decisions were made in a matter-of-fact manner and the mothers displayed little anxiety about following their own wishes. In the majority of cases formula was added within the first six weeks.

The reasons for adding formula and for weaning in this group were similar to those given by mothers who found weaning distressing, but the women simply experienced less ambivalence and anguish as they made their decision. The overall tone conveyed by these mothers was one of confidence and pragmatism. They were not, however, spared feelings of regret and sadness when they weaned. This was particularly true for women who enjoyed breast feeding and who stopped primarily because they were returning to work. Carol, for example, found that she was 'obsessed' with continuing to breast feed even though the baby came to prefer the bottle. She persevered with breast and bottle until it was quite evident that her baby preferred the bottle. She reluctantly weaned him earlier than she would have wished. So while she did not agonize over her decision she still felt distress and sadness.

All but two of the women who weaned without major distress had previous experience with breast feeding. It was evident from their comments that their prior experiences had realistically tempered their expectations and had helped them clarify how they would deal with issues that arose over the course of breast feeding. The air of confidence of these women contrasted sharply with the uncertainty and sense of inadequacy expressed by women who found weaning distressing. Perhaps the experienced mother gained confidence that enabled her to cope more easily with decisions related to breast feeding. The two mothers who had breast fed previously but who were included in the distressed group both had babies who were colicky, so their previous experience was of little value to them in coping with this new situation.

CHAPTER THIRTEEN

Reasons for Early Weaning

The reasons for weaning prior to four months fell into four categories. The first category, 'culture shock,' encompasses women who stopped because a combination of factors created a situation that was unfamiliar and often shocking. The second category, 'self-concern,' includes women who weaned primarily because breast feeding interfered with meeting their own needs. A third group, 'medical advice,' includes women who supplemented on the advice of their physician and subsequently weaned. The last category, 'paid employment,' included those who weaned because they were returning to work.

Culture Shock

Approximately one-third of the women who weaned prior to four months referred to a constellation of factors that influenced their decision to supplement and to wean. All but one of these women were first-time mothers and all found the arrival of a new baby overwhelming. There were so many changes and factors to contend with that mothers were reeling in the face of them. For all mothers, and perhaps especially first-time mothers, this post-partum period could be a time of tumultuous emotions and vulnerability as the realities of motherhood unfolded. Within this context a mother might cope easily with any one or two factors but an accumulation of factors could build to the point where 'something had to give.' Often, what gave was breast feeding because the mode of feeding was one area over which the mother could exercise some control. The factors that singly or in combination appeared to tip the balance toward a decision to wean are described below.

Maintaining Previous Life-style

Women who liked to be 'on the go' or who liked to manage their lives in an organized and predictable fashion could find the early post-partum period frustrating. They spoke of the difficulty of managing to be showered and dressed before noon. They described their homes as being in 'chaos' and meals as 'hodgepodge.' Betty spoke of her frustrations: 'When you don't have a chance to get dressed before ten o'clock in the morning because the baby needs stuff and you're still in your nightgown, that bothers me too. You know I like to be organized and start the day and go from there. Then you see your house deteriorating around you – dust, your husband coming home. You haven't had a chance to get dinner started and anxieties build up. They may seem like small things but they're huge and they bother you.'

Breast feeding was viewed as a major deterrent to being organized because it is time consuming, can only be done by the mother, and requires her to be in one place and to be attending to only one thing. Some women believed they were temperamentally unsuited to such an activity. Ann commented: 'The baby nursed really well right from the very beginning. If I analysed it I would say there's a chance that I'd be able to successfully breast feed, if somebody locked me in a cupboard without any external stimuli at all. I'm very susceptible to my environment and I'm just too interested in everything that's going on. I am not one that can sit and do nothing. It wasn't important enough to me to want to do that at all. I just felt, let's get on with it.'

Fatigue, especially in the early weeks, played a major role in a mother's inability to be as organized as she might wish to be. Jane, who felt like a 'zombie' because of spending her days sleeping and feeding, discussed fatigue:

I don't think I was prepared for so much fatigue. I find I just put off things. I've had ironing sitting for two weeks. The trouble is you wake up in the morning full of ideas, that I'll get this done, I'll get that done but in an hour or two I'm ready to just go to sleep. It's hard for someone who's always been really busy to accept that I'm just not doing anything with my life but sleeping. It's funny how that seems to be connected to the breast feeding. If it was bottle feeding I wouldn't be so tired.

A number of the women who stopped breast feeding early looked back and decided that they had attempted to do too much too soon, and that this effort had contributed to their lack of success with breast feeding. Carlson (1976) described the compulsion that some women experience after birth to complete a series of tasks that will prove they are normal and whole again. They are handicapped, of course, by their recovery from childbirth and by fatigue, but nevertheless may feel driven to return to their pre-pregnancy life-style.

Physical Discomfort

A variety of factors contributed to physical discomfort, which, in turn, contributed to some women's decision to stop breast feeding. Painful breasts are frequently cited in studies that examine reasons for early cessation (Feinstein, Berkelhamer, Gruszka, Wong, and Carey 1986; Gunn 1984; Martin 1978; Yeung et al. 1981). Sore nipples and engorgement were one source of discomfort in this study. In one case bleeding nipples were a major factor in introducing formula. In another instance a woman had a blocked duct at five weeks post-partum that was so painful that she decided to wean. For a third woman, the pain of sore nipples was a constant aggravation in the early weeks and was a significant factor in the introduction of a supplement. As time passed that problem lessened (and others emerged), but the pain triggered the first step of formula introduction, which, in her case, ultimately encouraged early weaning. Leaking breasts were also annoying. This alone was insufficient reason to stop breast feeding but many of these women disliked dripping breasts and going without clothes to air their nipples. Another factor was a concern for personal appearance, which was frequently linked to weight. Women often disliked the look of their bodies at this stage and felt overweight and bloated. Like leaking, appearance was generally not enough of a concern to be a major factor but was perceived as an additional burden associated with breast feeding because mothers believed it was an inappropriate time to diet. Gruis (1977), Mercer (1981), and Russell (1974) all found that personal appearance was a major concern of new mothers. Reconciling their postpartum bodies with their idealized body images was a major component of the 'grief work' that Mercer (1981) described as a part of adjusting to motherhood.

Baby's Reponse to Breast Feeding

A major factor in the introduction of formula for all the women who suffered from culture shock was their infants' response to breast feeding. It was disconcerting for the mother when the baby pulled back from the breast and cried or resisted taking the nipple. This was perceived as rejection and was unexpected and traumatic for the mother. Julie had a Caesarian birth and it was three days before the baby was breast fed. He did not adapt well to breast feeding. Julie described the baby's reactions to both breast and bottle after three weeks of sustained effort at breast feeding: 'He was the same hysterical feeder that he had been the week before. The fact that the milk didn't come instantly put him off totally. He was hardly sucking at all, but he was there – just totally miserable. Then I'd give him a bottle and he'd be fine and happy and quite content. I persisted with that for the week and then nothing changed. He certainly didn't get any better.

I would just get him to the breast and he would shriek and scream.'

In Julie's case the baby had clearly developed a preference for the bottle over the breast. In other instances the cause of the baby's upset was much less clear but the behaviour was similar. Sometimes the baby was diagnosed as having colic. While this labelled the problem, the baby's unhappiness during and after feeding was still upsetting. In all cases, a shift to formula was an option that mothers believed must be tried, although this did not resolve the colic or necessarily lead to weaning.

In the majority of cases where the baby was clearly unhappy, the mother questioned whether she was producing an adequate quantity of milk. All the mothers in this group commented at one point or another that they thought that their supply was probably inadequate. Despite these comments they did not conclude that low milk supply was the source of the problem. These women were all knowledgeable about the supply/demand principle and the factors that negatively influence supply. Women who supplemented soon after birth or whose babies did not feed well or frequently enough were aware that their breasts would need more stimulation in order to increase the overall volume. The mothers were also aware of the links between emotional stress, fatigue, and milk production. In many instances they speculated that their supply was low because they were exhausted, angry, tense, or anxious. They hoped that relaxation and frequent feedings would improve their supply. In some cases the volume of milk increased but other factors became more critical in the decision to wean. In other cases mothers were unwilling to face the stresses that accompanied increasing the milk supply (frequent feedings, sore nipples, limits on mobility, etc.).

As was seen in chapter 6, mothers frequently attributed their uncertainty about the adequacy of their milk to the fact that they could not see how much milk the baby was taking. Some of the mothers, who had worried about their supply and had assumed that they were producing insufficient amounts, questioned this assumption once they began to wean. As they nursed less often many quickly experienced breast engorgement and concluded they had more milk than they originally thought.

It is interesting that most studies that examine the factors influencing breast feeding rarely cite the baby's temperament as an important component. Presumably, when the baby cries or is unhappy the mother attributes the problem to breast milk rather than simply to the baby's temperament. Most studies ask mothers why they stop. However, in one study on early cessation the investigators (Loughlin, Clapp-Channing, Gehlbach, Pollard, and McCutchen 1985) also asked nursery nurses to assess the babies with regard to how much they cried, their feeding behaviour, their personalities, and the nurses' prediction of future breast-feeding problems. It turned out that factors statistically associated with early weaning included the nurses' ratings of excessive crying, a demanding personality, trouble with feeding, and predicted problems. These findings suggest that the baby's temperament may play an important role in the success or failure of breast feeding.

Unmet Expectations

Another factor contributing to a readiness to stop breast feeding was the mother's disappointment about the quality of her interaction with the baby during feeding and her recognition that bottle feeding was a viable alternative. The disappointment was often fuelled by the fact that the reality of breast feeding did not measure up to pre-birth expectations. Eleanor was a case in point: 'One of the things that has really surprised me about the breast-feeding experience is that I don't really feel that it's such a wonderfully romantic thing. Maybe it's because of the problems I've had. You read about this incredible warmth and closeness, but I can hold her close and cuddle her while I'm giving her the bottle and get the same kind of feelings.'

Many women had expected an immediate bonding to occur

with breast feeding but they learned that these two things were not necessarily linked. Julie's baby was so unhappy breast feeding that she decided to stop: 'All of the reasons that I had wanted to breast feed were not holding. He was bonding much better to me with the bottle and we would cuddle up. It was a chore to breast feed. It was really me saying, "I want to breast feed and we're going to do it." And he wasn't getting anything to speak of. So I decided that I wasn't really getting what I wanted out of it at all. And I wasn't seeing him getting anything out of it either. It just didn't seem to be the right thing.'

Betty spoke about discovering the reality of breast feeding: 'Everybody said it comes so naturally but it doesn't. It takes a lot to get to feel comfortable with them and to know them. It has just been hard coping with the reality or just the delusion of everything coming so naturally and falling into place. That's not necessarily true. I guess I had a fairly romantic idea of breast feeding and when the reality hits, it has its drawbacks.'

In the end, a few mothers in our study concluded that bottle feeding was as satisfactory as breast feeding or that the method of feeding was not necessarily a major factor in determining the quality of the relationship they developed with their baby.

Personal Needs

Following the birth of a baby most mothers find there are major changes in the amount of time available to meet their personal needs or other responsibilities. The importance of these needs was sometimes a factor in deciding to wean early. For example, Elizabeth concluded after a brief period of breast feeding: 'It is just wrong for me and I have no intention of being tied down.' Betty also discovered that insufficient time for herself was a major disadvantage of breast feeding:

That's also a big change when you know you can't even have dinner together anymore. I really resent that. Don eats, then I eat, and I can't stand that because I really enjoy that time for us to talk. You live, eat, and breathe baby all day. I feel strongly about motherhood but I feel that I need to be me as well. I need adult conversation and I am just not that child oriented that I want to lose my own identity. I want an hour or so to just curl up, read a newspaper or book, or put my feet up. I want her fed. I want her happy but let me do my thing for an hour.

Lack of Knowledge/Skills

Many women frequently spoke about their uncertainty about how to breast feed, about judging the adequacy of their milk supply, and about the meaning of the baby's crying or pushing away from the breast, and demands for frequent feedings. Some mothers believed that they would 'know' all these things if they were adequate mothers. Not knowing and the accompanying feelings of inadequacy tended to undermine their confidence. Bottle feeding was an attractive alternative because if the baby was not satisfied by the formula, the dissatisfaction and rejection would not reflect so personally on the mother.

None of the above factors, in isolation, was likely to result in a decision to wean. However, when a number of factors converged over a short period of time the likelihood of weaning increased. This pattern of converging factors is similar to the findings of Sjolin et al. (1979) in their prospective study of the breast-feeding experience of 146 Swedish women. They found, as did we, that 'each individual mother reacted in her own special way to motherhood and to difficult situations' (p. 523). Likewise, they noted that although there was a wide variety of reasons for early weaning there seemed to be a convergence of problems that ultimately led to early weaning. They concluded that 'sometimes several problems in combination seemed to form the causative factor, and in some cases there was a chain of more or less harmless events that sooner or later resulted in lactation crisis or weaning' (p. 526).

The nature of the concerns experienced by the women in

our study is similar to those reported by Chapman et al. (1985), Grassley and Davis (1978), Gruis (1977), Sjolin et al. (1979), and Summer and Fritsch (1977). Concerns about actual feeding problems were inextricably linked to other issues in the mother's life such as fatigue, body discomfort and body image, social support (or lack of), role adjustments, and self-confidence.

Jane's decision to stop breast feeding illustrates the convergence of a variety of concerns. In her final interview she reviewed the contributing factors:

Right from the very first day when I nursed him I probably left him on the breast too long and he really chomped at the nipple. That took a long time to heal. So I didn't get off to a great start. When I started to have problems I just figured this is the beginning and it will get better and what I found was that it really didn't get better. I was in pain while he was eating and that was causing a lot of unhappiness – he doesn't even want it. I wasn't allowing him to feed long enough because I was uncomfortable. The worst feeds were in the middle of the night when I was tired and frustrated. I'd be sitting there thinking, 'What am I doing this for?' I really started to build up some resentment to him and then I started to feel that I was lashing out at my husband.

One of the problems that I had in breast feeding is that sometimes I probably put too much on my plate. In the first month I really shouldn't have been so busy. What happens is that the breast feeding is taking longer and I have someone coming over, or am organized to do something and I'm trying to do two things at once. I was somewhat unrealistic about the whole thing of how much work the baby is.

It's very hard to just sort of let everything else just go. I was reading a home magazine talking about some superwomen who have dinner parties and carry on a full-time job and are new mothers. It's just overwhelming and I think that that is part of the problem. You've just got to be perfect.

The few times that I had given him a bottle, I really enjoyed it. I started to think about why am I doing this and is this worth it? Is this good for both of us? What are the benefits versus the non-benefits? I didn't want to be a quitter.

Because of problems related to the pregnancy we haven't had intercourse in four months. I started to relax, we talked about it, and I decided the time was right to have intercourse again. My whole body was very scared and tight and sensitive. I did partly blame it on the breast feeding because my breasts were so sore and big and so full. I really couldn't enjoy the usual positions that we enjoy.

I wanted to get back to my pre-pregnant shape and feel more potent, more normal again. I just felt I owed it to myself not to be a martyr.

I wasn't getting these lovely feelings that I read about and thought that I would get [from] breast feeding. I was missing a lot of the closeness that first few weeks because I was unhappy and was really in pain. So I just decided that I would make the decision to stop. I've sort of set as my goals that I would like to have him pretty well all weaned when we go away on our holidays. I really do need to have a relaxing holiday.

Self-concern

Just under one-third of the mothers who stopped breast feeding prior to four months did so for reasons primarily related to their own well-being. These women placed a priority on maintaining an appropriate balance between the needs of their child or children and their own needs. All but one of these women had breast fed before and were therefore quite clear about how they wished to handle breast feeding. Kim said she stopped breast feeding at six weeks because of her own personality. She claimed she 'felt like a cow,' 'looked horrible,' and was on a 'short fuse' while breast feeding. She stopped for what she termed selfish reasons because she wanted to fit into her clothes and because she wanted to be out, without the baby, for longer periods of time. Routines were important to her and she concluded that breast feeding was not a viable option because she 'couldn't handle the thought of not having everything organized.' She saw organization as the key to ensuring time away from the children.

Cheryl was breast feeding for the second time even though she really disliked it. She could not understand why it was so revered. She did not like being at the 'demand of the child,' did not find breast feeding relaxing, and had to 'fend off' her two-year-old while breast feeding the baby. Her appearance and general comfort were important to her and she wanted to be able to diet. She said, 'You have to look good in order to have a lot of confidence in yourself.' Despite her strong views Cheryl breast fed for eleven weeks because her baby disliked the formula and found breast feeding soothing. Cheryl actually switched paediatricians because the first paediatrician wanted her to continue with breast milk since the baby vomited the formula.

Another mother introduced formula five days post-partum and by two months was breast feeding only twice a day. During her first week at home things had 'fallen apart,' because she had no support and did not know who to call. She had recently experienced a tragic death in her family and was providing support to others. Her response to the situation was a very pragmatic one: 'At that point I wasn't in any mood to let Jason rule my time.' She also made reference to not wishing to be a 'slave to breast feeding.'

Yet another mother with three children found it frustrating to breast feed even though she enjoyed it. She had many visitors and would not breast feed publicly. She also said: 'I wouldn't tell anybody to breast feed, full time. Not 100 per cent. I just can't go for it. Everybody needs a little bit of time for themselves especially if you have other children.'

Medical Advice

Four women weaned early because of medical advice. One

woman lived in an impoverished and unstable home situation and was physically abused. She had trouble getting enough to eat. Although her physician had encouraged breast feeding it became obvious that her milk supply was inadequate and she was advised to stop.

In the second instance the baby simply refused the breast, failed to gain weight, and was therefore weaned within four weeks of birth.

In the other two cases the babies were fussy and unhappy but both mothers were stunned when their physicians recommended supplementing breast feeding with formula. Jennifer introduced formula at four weeks on the doctor's advice and continued, with much ambivalence, to give mixed feedings of bottle and breast until twelve weeks post-partum. Her uncertainty about how to feed her baby was fuelled by his colicky nature and ultimately she decided to settle on one form of feeding.

Laurie, whose experience with her physician was described in chapter 5, initally refused to follow her doctor's advice to supplement with formula and embarked on a course of increasing her milk supply by pumping, getting extra rest, and drinking more fluids. As well, she selected a new doctor. However, the seeds of doubt that had been planted earlier began to grow. By the tenth week she felt she had come to 'a turn in the road' because she believed her son needed more than she could provide. She introduced cereal and fruit even though she knew her doctor would disapprove. In the face of pressure from other family members she concluded she had made a 'terrible mistake.' She then stopped the solid food, instead offering formula when she thought he needed it. Over the next three weeks she weaned him completely. She was anticipating a return to work and concluded there was little point in pumping once she was feeding formula.

Paid Employment

Two of the women who weaned prematurely did so primarily

because they returned to work. Carol went back on a part-time basis four weeks after the baby's birth and intended to make her decision about weaning in response to how things worked out. Initially she took the baby to work with her but by eleven weeks she began to leave him at home and pumped milk for him. The baby very quickly came to prefer a bottle to the breast and Carol regretfully weaned him.

Diane had intended to stop breast feeding when she returned to work. With sadness, she introduced formula at eleven weeks and the baby was weaned by the time she started work.

Many other women returned to work some time after the four-month mark. These women were fortunate enough to have employers who allowed longer, although unpaid, maternity leaves.

For some first-time mothers the realities of the responsibilities of motherhood and the difficulties encountered in breast feeding led to a questioning of their feeding choice and ultimately to a decision to wean early. Women who had breast fed before, and who had had mixed reactions then, were prepared to try again. They were quite clear about their priority to balance their own needs with those of their new babies. If the balance was upset they were prepared to stop breast feeding. A smaller number of women weaned on the advice of their physician or because of a return to the labour force.

The decision to wean could be accompanied by a good deal of ambivalence and distress on the part of the mother. In the face of a strong belief in the value of breast feeding and high expectations about the influence of breast feeding on the quality of the relationship with the baby, it could be disconcerting to contemplate stopping.

CHAPTER FOURTEEN

Weaning between Four Months and One Year

The decision to wean was much simpler once the baby reached four to five months of age. Approximately one-third of the women that we followed one year weaned between four and twelve months post-partum. Forty-two per cent of this group were still breast feeding at one year. Women were three times more likely to wean between seven and twelve months than they were between four and seven months. Many expressed a preference to wean directly to cow's milk in a cup, and so avoid formula and bottles. The pattern of distressed weaning described in chapter 12 was rarely evident after four months because most mothers believed they had given their child a good start. Of the women who weaned after four months just over one-half stopped primarily because of their own needs, either physical or emotional. One-quarter stopped because they were returning to work and did not wish to combine the two activities. The remainder weaned because of factors related to the baby.

Weaning Because of the Mother's Needs

There were many personal factors that influenced the decision to stop breast feeding. A number of mothers weaned because of their desire for more freedom. For example, one mother, whose baby had refused to take a bottle, felt the strain of being the only person who could feed her infant. She felt tied down but had continued breast feeding for over seven months because her baby had a congenital heart defect and she wished to spare him unnecessary anxiety. A number of mothers wanted to travel without the baby. In some instances the baby accompanied the mother but travelling was thought to be simpler if the baby was bottle fed.

Physical well-being also influenced when weaning occurred. One mother who developed arthritis prolonged breast feeding as long as she could but finally weaned when she could no longer manage the pain without medication. Another mother was pregnant and concluded that trying to feed a baby and cope with pregnancy was just too much. The desire to lose weight was also a contributing factor. Some women were fed up with clothes that didn't fit and 'flabby' bodies. Conversely, another woman attributed her weight loss and poor food intake to breast feeding. She concluded, 'It was just too hard on me.'

Although fatigue was less of a factor in a decision to wean at this time than it was prior to four months, it was still significant for a few women. Estelle, who had two other small children, weaned at nine and a half months. Fatigue was an important component: 'I was not at all ready for him to wean. I knew I was getting tired and the milk supply was getting lower. I could feel it. I was afraid it might happen and I didn't want it to. But it did.'

Roslyn, a single mother, had numerous reasons for wanting to wean. She loved breast feeding but by five months she was tired and wanted to make a number of changes: 'I've stopped nursing her now because it's got to be too much for me. I'm not losing weight fast enough and its draining! I didn't really have what it took to carry on. It was totally for my convenience, not for hers. I needed to have a little bit more freedom in what I could do. I could not continue my life as I knew it. It's wonderful being a mother but you need a little bit of time for mum, too. You have to remember that you have needs, too.'

Weaning Because of Work

By the one-year point almost half the women in the study group were employed outside the home, on either a full-time or part-time basis. One-third of these had weaned their babies prior to four months post-partum. Of the remaining women, one-third weaned their babies because of returning to work. They usually planned the weaning in advance and allowed at least a month to complete the process. The other two-thirds continued to breast feed and work outside the home. In most cases they breast fed their babies in the morning before work and before bedtime and left formula for the other feedings. Women who worked part time had more flexibility and could offer more breast feeds per day.

Statistically, our study findings indicated that women who were not employed outside the home breast fed longer than those women who were employed full time or part time.

The women who stopped because of returning to work did not discuss in detail the reasons for their decisions. They simply stated that they wished to wean the baby before starting work. Those who continued to breast feed while working did not encounter major difficulties. No doubt by four months their milk supply was well established and they had experience in mastering minor crises. Auerbach and Guss (1984), in a study of work and breast feeding, found that infant weaning prior to one year of age is highest when the mother returns to full-time employment before the infant is sixteen weeks old. This age factor was more important than the number of hours worked per week. Although it is possible for employed mothers to continue breast feeding, the onus is clearly on the mother to make it work. Few employers offer any incentives that would make breast feeding easy for the working mother. Following a recent survey of 100 of the most profitable companies in the United States drawn from the Fortune 500 list, Moore and Jansa (1987) were unable to document generalized support for breast-feeding mothers. They concluded that there is an urgent need for the public and health professionals to lobby for programs to support breast feeding in the work place. Such measures would include extended maternity leave, day-care benefits, private facilities with refrigerators in the work place for milk expression or feeding the baby, and enhanced family-oriented employee health care.

Weaning Because of the Baby

Another important factor that contributed to a decision to stop breast feeding was changes in the baby. Two or three mothers decided to wean because their babies' teeth were coming in and they did not want to risk being bitten. A few babies lost interest in breast feeding. Estelle, who was described above, weaned primarily because of fatigue and the decrease in her milk supply. However, she also believed that her son was ready: 'I don't think it was just my milk supply being low because it wasn't low enough that it would have caused him to quit. He had enough offers of liquid otherwise so that nutritionally he was taken care of. So if it was comfort sucking that he wanted, it was available and he just didn't need me anymore.'

Other women reported the same thing. The baby just appeared indifferent to the breast: 'He's about 99 per cent weaned. It happened really quickly and it was basically his decision. It was really strange. About two and a half weeks ago he started this business where, except for the morning feeding, he'd nurse for a second, then become disinterested and look around for ten minutes and become distracted by absolutely anything. Getting him to nurse a complete feeding was impossible.'

Some studies have reported high rates of infant-initiated weaning between five and nine months (Clark and Harmon 1983; Waletzky 1977, 1979). It has been suggested that this is more likely a result of cognitive and physical growth spurts that cause the baby to take a greater interest in activities other than breast feeding than an indicator of a desire to wean

(Clark and Harmon 1983). None the less, if the mother is ready to wean then, it may provide a mutually acceptable time to do so.

The baby's age also had a bearing on cessation. The mother whose arthritis caused her to stop breast feeding also commented: 'At this point I think she should be doing more grown up things than breast feeding. I associate it more with babies.' Her baby was approximately ten months old at the time. A few others had planned to breast feed until their infants were a year old and then stop. This point of view is typified by the following: 'I tend to feel that once a child is walking, has teeth, and is able to eat, it's time to start weaning them. I think a year is that cut-off point.'

Sometimes there was no particular reason to wean; it was simply that the first birthday signalled a reasonable time to stop.

The Process of Weaning

Most of the women who weaned their babies between four months and one year did so gradually. They believed it was better for their babies and themselves. Cynthia described how she stopped breast feeding:

I started slowly in January. I would nurse him morning and night still. I bottle fed him two ounces and then I nursed him. The next night I would do the same. Then the next night three ounces of bottle and three minutes of nursing. I slowly paced it so that I was only nursing him maybe two minutes and six ounces of a bottle. I think it was for me, too. I didn't want to give up giving him the breast and I thought this was the best way to do it. So I cut down slowly. Then in February, it was a Sunday, we came back from my mum's and I thought, 'I'm just going to give him a bottle.' I gave him a bottle and told him it was time to go to bed and put him to bed and nothing, no problem. Monday a.m. he woke up and I offered him a bottle instead of the breast and he had it. Then that night I gave him a bottle and then it was just one of those things where the next morning I gave him a bottle.

Other women substituted a bottle for an entire feeding. Lana's description was typical: 'She was about six and a half months because she was able to go on cow's milk then. That's the first time she would accept a bottle. The first couple of weeks I just tried to give her a bottle a day. Then she was taking two a day and then three. She got down to about one breast feed a day. And she stopped that when she was about nine and a half to ten months old.'

She believed that the baby's readiness was an important factor: 'She weaned herself. I didn't have to do anything. There was no problem changing to a bottle. She did it very gradually. No fighting about. She didn't even miss it. There was over four months from the introduction of a bottle to the last snack on the breast.'

As she was weaning Lorna vascillated on her decision: 'Sometimes I would just think, "Oh, forget it," and suddenly nurse again. Eventually I just decided, "No, I've got to stop completely," and I gave her bottles.'

Some attempted to wean more quickly. This could cause problems, as Tracey discovered. She had tried to wean her son earlier but he had refused to take a bottle. When she tried the second time, six weeks later, the baby took the bottle easily: 'I weaned him faster than I intended. I did it over a period of about ten days. I thought while the going is good I will keep going. The last couple of days of weaning the left breast was so engorged I was in pure agony. From the physical discomfort I had I know I did it too quickly. I never in my life experienced such pain. I don't think giving birth was this painful.'

Christina weaned somewhat less quickly and had no problems: 'Weaning took about three weeks altogether. I intended to do it a lot more gradually but it just didn't work. I guess the milk supply went down. Then I found it easy giving her a bottle. I didn't have any engorgement at all.'

Mothers' Feelings about Weaning

Over half the mothers commented on how they felt about weaning. Feelings ranged from satisfaction to ambivalence to sadness. One-quarter of the mothers spoke positively about breast feeding ending, believing there would be fewer demands on them. One mother commented that because of weaning she was starting to feel her best again. Another said that she had not had strong feelings about breast feeding and therefore did not have strong feelings about stopping. Tracey was happy to have stopped. She relished the freedom and the opportunity to get her figure back: 'By the time he was weaned I was quite relieved. It was nice. It was as if he was ready also. After he was weaned I went to a shopping plaza and fed him a bottle. I sat there and thought, "This is just fantastic." Now the most important thing is for me to wear things that you can see my waist. It's important for me to get back to my own figure.'

Although weaning was not Christina's preference she accepted it with equanimity:

I don't have regrets about weaning. If I had my druthers I'd stay home a bit longer – maybe 'til she was a year old, and I'd keep nursing her. But it's good for me to go back to work and financially I have to. For those reasons I don't have any regrets at all about weaning her. And she's had just short of six months at the breast and I think that's pretty good. It's made it nice for me because I have so much freedom now, all of a sudden. Psychologically it's really different, too, because now I'm just back to being me.

More frequently, mothers were ambivalent about weaning. They were relieved to be rid of the responsibility but saddened by the loss of that special form of nurturing. Weaning was a marker event. It signified the baby's growing independence and some women felt sad that the first phase of infancy was over:

It just means that she's no longer a baby. She doesn't need me any more in that way. That's really hard.

He is my last child. It's the last time I get to do this. I wasn't ready for it to end.

I stopped two weeks ago. It's a bit of a let-down. It gave me a sense of finality. I'm not going to be able to change my mind. There is a sense of loss. It feels awkward, strange, that I wasn't nursing him. I miss the closeness and the convenience and the less mechanical aspects. I still find the bottle a foreign object whereas the breast is much more personal.

A few women found that weaning was far more traumatic than they had expected. The trauma centred around their perception that the baby's loss of interest in breast feeding was a form of rejection. Fiona, who weaned at five months, primarily because the baby lost interest, was devastated. She was surprised by her feelings because she had intended to initiate weaning in less than a month in any event. She described her reactions.

I'm finding it really difficult to give up. It's the separation. I had so many feelings both positive and negative about breast feeding. I was feeling really tied down and things like that. One would think that I'd welcome him wanting to wean. But it's funny, that's not how I feel at all. I thought, 'He's got to wean sometime. He can't stay at your breast forever. This is when it's best for him so just do it.' But it's funny how I felt so desperate. I even started reading about relactation. I had planned to breast feed until six months. I felt that I had worked through the beginning awful stages so with that I was going to hit six months and be really proud of myself. Then I would wean him gradually and nurse him nights only until he was about a year. When he wanted to wean it was traumatic. There's no other word for it. It was this rejection I was feeling from my son – his putting mummy aside and wanting a bottle. I felt I was losing the bond. I went through that whole thing of 'now he doesn't need me anymore!' That was a really heavy thing. Now anybody could take care of him! In retrospect I'm glad he did it so I wouldn't have to. Because if he wanted to continue nursing I couldn't wean him. I'd feel like I was depriving him of something he really loved.

The rates of weaning found in this study should serve as a

standard for what can be achieved in the Canadian setting. At six and twelve months, 74 and 42 per cent, respectively, of our sample were still breast feeding. By four months, the rewards outweighed the difficulties and women had the opportunity to relax and enjoy breast feeding. When the time to wean arrived they could do it in a way that was satisfactory to both themselves and the baby.

PART FIVE

Support Networks

Social support is considered crucial to the success of breast feeding efforts. Recommendations about enhancing support for breast-feeding women are prominently featured in all the major position papers on breast feeding. An in-depth analysis of 141 articles on breast feeding found that support was the major factor discussed in all articles (Harrison, More, and Prowse 1985). In another review on support and breast feeding, Cronenwett and Reinhardt (1987) reported that persons the mothers viewed as influential varied with their ethnic and socio-economic status. The male partner and friends were important for Anglo-Americans, the subjects' mothers were important for Hispanics, and close friends were important for black women. The authors also reported that women who have friends who have breast fed, support from family and friends, and access to information sources are likely to breast feed longer than women who do not have these types of support. Despite the importance placed on support there is surprisingly little research that elucidates the actual dynamics of social support and examines the management of breast feeding within the family context.

In this section of the book the various situations in which mothers look for support with breast feeding are examined. Unfortunately, support is not always forthcoming. In part three, 'The Realities of Breast Feeding,' women spoke of their experiences in the hospital, with their physicians, and with family members, and they highlighted the problems. Their comments were useful because by turning them around it is possible to see what can be done to help women to have a more positive experience of breast feeding.

Institutional arrangements – whether in the hospital, in the physician's office, in the family, or in the community – need to be examined and changed if women are to have an easier time. Recommendations for change are interspersed in the text of the chapters in this section. The concluding chapter, in part six, sums up the social influences on women's experiences of breast feeding.

CHAPTER FIFTEEN

Breast Feeding in the Hospital

During their hospital stay women wanted emotional support, help, and practical advice on breast feeding to get off to a good start. Almost all the women interviewed commented on the degree of support they received from hospital staff. The majority spoke positively, although briefly, about what they considered supportive behaviour. Comments like the following were typical: 'The nurses are fabulous. They're fabulous. They're very attentive to your personal needs. They're fantastic. Had it not been for the nurses being so good I'm sure I wouldn't have been feeding as well as I have been. They're just always there to help whenever you need them.' / 'The nursing staff this time has been phenomenal. I've got nothing but praise for them.'

Mothers appreciated it when nurses offered suggestions in a way that respected the mother's right to decide what to do:

The staff has been really good, even the one nurse that I had the argument with this morning. She was telling me that when he wakes up I must actually insist that he take both breasts at each feeding even though he's sleepy. But even she ended it up saying, "This is our recommendation, you do what you want." You know, she's pretty strong with her recommendation but she still gave room, which was really kind of nice. The vast majority of the nurses have been absolutely wonderful.

Having some autonomy in the hospital was important. One mother said, 'They really left me to do what I wanted.' Another said, 'The hospital was really good about respecting my wishes.'

The importance of nurses taking a positive attitude was also emphasized. Mothers commented favourably about nurses who expressed confidence about their abilities to breast feed: 'The nurses were really good about helping with breast feeding. They were very encouraging and very positive.'

Women appreciated warmth and kindness as well. The new mother needed some mothering herself. Nurses were sometimes referred to as 'loving,' 'warm,' 'kind,' and 'comforting.' The following example illustrates a situation in which such attitudes were appreciated. In this instance the mother had had an argument with the nurses about her wish to be the person to feed glucose water to her baby. The argument had been resolved in the mother's favour but afterwards she had been upset. She described how the nurse handled this situation: 'The nurses were really kind. Sometimes you get very irritable when you're not feeling well and things are bothering you. Instead of the nurse reacting in a negative way, she said, "I'm sorry that you feel like that, dear. What can I do to make you more comfortable?"'

Approximately one-third of the women we interviewed were dissatisfied with their hospital experience. They spoke in more detail and used examples to illustrate behaviour they found bothersome. The common element running through all of the negative comments was a lack of effective communication. Five categories of difficulties arose.

Confusion about Hospital Policy

Common to many women's experience was the failure of staff to communicate hospital policy on issues of importance to mothers. These issues included the opportunity for demand feeding, the use of supplemental formula, water, or glucose water, rooming in, and feeding policies, especially night feedings for mothers who had had Caesarian sections. There were numerous examples of problems and confusion arising because mothers did not know what the policy was or the degree to which the policy was flexible. This confusion upset the mother at a time when she was already feeling emotionally charged. Mothers felt forced into confrontations because of their uncertainty about what was happening with their babies. Withholding the baby so the mother could rest and giving supplemental bottles were particularly upsetting policies. The following excerpts convey the nature of the mothers' concerns and the intensity of their feelings in the days just following birth:

They forgot to bring him to me for the 5:30 or 6 feed. I called down to the station and said, 'Where is he?' 'Oh, he wasn't marked down to be brought to you. So, he's been fed.' I panicked. 'Do you mean they've given him some formula or something?' I was really upset. I marched down to the nursery and that was not easy as I discovered I had a very uncomfortable episiotomy. I said, 'Give me my baby. I'm taking him out of here.' They'd only given him water it turns out but still he wasn't thirsty because he'd had water.

I woke up about 7 and my milk had come in so I buzzed down to the nurse and I said, 'Well, what happened? Why didn't you bring my baby for a feeding?' They said, 'Oh, you were asleep. We didn't want to wake you up.' So I was really upset about that because there I was, finally with my milk, and they didn't bring him!

I hadn't seen her since she was born. It was almost a whole day. I wanted to know where my baby was. They said, 'The baby was born by C-section and we think that you need your rest. Because you had a big operation you shouldn't be up yet.' I started to cry because I thought she was starving and she had no food, and my poor baby was going to die undernourished. They thought I was crazy. They said,

'We're going to give her glucose water.' I said 'I want to give it to her.' So they put up a bit of a fuss and eventually they took me down to the nursery, closed the little curtain around me, and I fed the baby.

Apparently they did give him formula in the hospital, which I didn't find out until Saturday morning when I was discharged. That concerned me because I thought, 'Well, if they've been giving him more at night-time than I knew about then perhaps I don't have enough milk right now to satisfy him because he's been getting a couple more ounces than I knew about.' That was quite concerning to me. I did say something to the nurse about it and she was quite defensive. She said, 'What do you expect us to do, feed them water?' I said, 'I certainly don't but I left a message that I wanted to be wakened to feed him.' She said that they were very concerned about me. I was very concerned that they would do that because I really wanted to breast feed him. So it was once again their making decisions about me and what I need. I know I needed rest, but I also knew what I could do.

Hospital procedures should be clearly communicated so women know in advance what to expect. They can then temper their expectations or try to have procedures adapted to suit their own needs. Ultimately, hospital staff must respect women's ability to make decisions for themselves.

But How Do I Breast Feed?

Mothers needed to be taught how to breast feed at the time of the baby's first feeding. They complained, however, that there was a lack of information and practical advice at this time. The lack of guidance with early breast-feeding efforts left some women feeling abandoned by the hospital staff. Four mothers' descriptions of their first feeding experiences follow:

The nurse just kind of plopped the baby in my arms. I said, 'Hey, wait a minute.' I wasn't sure of what to do.

Breast Feeding in the Hospital 151

They didn't tell me anything! They just shoved me with my baby and said, 'Here you go.' If it wasn't for the girl beside me, I wouldn't have known how long to do it.

I wish they had given me more personalized instruction on breast feeding. They took a lot for granted. They didn't tell me that there is a special way to hold the baby, that when you take the baby off, to put your finger in the side of it's mouth so it releases the suction. I think that's what started everything going bad because the nipple got so sore. I really wish that they had gone through nipple care. When they brought her in the nurse said. 'Have you ever breast fed before?' I said, 'No.' It was a matter of like two minutes. She said, 'Well you just hold the baby up to your breast and point the nipple towards her mouth and that's it.' So the baby latched on and she left and that was it. They just leave you there.

We were all very disappointed by the teaching we got. Especially breast feeding. It was all just by osmosis. Nobody came in, for instance, and said, 'Do you need any help? This is how you breast feed.' You just had to cope on your own. I hadn't a clue how long I should do it. The third day, one of the head nurses came in and helped me a little bit. I was so engorged by then I couldn't really do it properly so I asked her myself for a nipple shield. We all had to just kind of do all our own care and figure out things by ourselves.

In some cases the nurses assumed that mothers were knowledgeable about breast feeding and therefore did not need any help, advice, or support: 'A lot of them ask you, "Is this your first baby or your second baby?" I said, "Well, it's my second one, but my first one is 16 years old. So they figure, "Well, she knows what she's doing." They just naturally assume that. I should have just turned around and said, "Yes, it is my first baby," and then they would have been a little more helpful with breast feeding. I guess he was so content in the nursery they figured he must be doing all right so they never bothered.'

To facilitate nursing, the skills required to breast feed need to be reviewed for experienced mothers as well as new mothers.

Mixed Messages

Mothers were frustrated when they received mixed messages from nursing staff about anything related to breast feeding:

This other nurse said to pump. The thing that really bugged me was that I got a different story from different nurses. One said, 'Don't pump.' Another one said, 'Pump.' As far as the professionals were concerned, I really got terrible support. I got conflicting opinions.

He was crying and it wasn't working. I didn't know what was wrong. I didn't know if I was feeding too little or too much. The student nurse was telling me I was feeding too little and another nurse came in and said, 'His bowels look loose, you're probably feeding him too much. When was the last time you fed him?' They were generally driving me crazy.

Conflicting advice, particularly during this early period of uncertainty, undermined all advice offered by staff because the mother had no way of determining which piece of advice was most appropriate.

Lack of Communication among Nurses

Lack of communication among nurses proved to be an aggravation for mothers. This was compounded when different nurses were assigned to mother care and infant care. Maternity nurses acted in the interest of the mother and nursery nurses in the interest of the baby. This division of responsibilities set up a situation in which mothers occasionally received different messages from the two sets of nurses. Also, the lack of communication between these two groups affected whether the mother's concerns were relayed to the appropriate staff person. The breakdown in communication that resulted from split responsibilities led to confusion, anger, and frustration at a time when mothers were trying to establish breast feeding.

A number of women talked about problems that arose as a consequence of communication breakdown between the two sets of nurses. Marla, for instance, recalled an incident when the baby was first brought to her: 'That first period if you've got a C-section is pretty difficult. And they don't offer advice for that. There's very little communication between nursery nurses and floor nurses. The first time they brought me Heidi, she actually brought her and plunked her down on my stomach, not knowing it was a section and I just about hit the roof with the pain.' Some hospitals have now switched to a system where one nurse takes care of both the mother and baby and this procedure should alleviate many of the communication problems.

There were a number of examples where mothers expected certain feeding procedures to be followed (for example, timing of feedings, night feedings, feeding of formula or glucose water) but encountered difficulties because the initial agreement between a nurse and a mother was not communicated to other nurses.

The failure to communicate messages between nurses happened even when they worked in the same area but on different shifts. The following example was not uncommon: 'I went over to the nursery and I had asked for him to come to me in the night on Monday night because I had already gotten my milk and I just wanted to get rid of it. So I went over there about 1. He was due to come at 1:30 and there was the nurse and he had just had three ounces of water. I could have cried. I was so uncomfortable. She said, "Oh, well." She got very defensive and said she had never gotten a message and that was that.'

Criticism

A number of women endured comments that called into

question their ability to nurse. At a time when mothers were coming to terms with a new skill and were coping with their new roles, these critical comments fuelled anxiety, anger, and a host of other negative emotions. A number of women recounted their reactions to criticism by hospital staff:

Last night I finally just yelled at a nurse. She says, 'You're feeding the baby too often.' I finally just had to be nasty almost to get her to realize I wasn't feeding too often and another nurse would come along and look and say, 'Oh, that's fine.'

There was another nurse who came when I was just getting started and said to me, 'Oh, your nipples are no good and you don't have enough milk.' She was so negative. She practically said to me, 'You're not going to be able to breast feed.'

I had asked my doctor beforehand about breast feeding on the delivery table and she discouraged me from doing it. She said, 'Wait until you're cleaned up and off on your own.' We went back to the labour room right after he was born. The nurse that had been with us was pretty A-1 but when I said, 'I'd like to nurse him,' she said, 'What do you want to do that for?' I was really disappointed. She said, 'Oh, he won't know anything about it yet.' She also said, 'You won't have anything for him, yet.'

Criticism introduced an air of pessimism and apprehension implying to women that they might be unable to breast feed.

The underlying causes of mothers' complaints about their hospital stay pointed to a number of factors that can influence the early days of breast feeding. Mothers need to understand what the hospital policies are and how much flexibility exists. They would benefit from having resource material on breast feeding and from participating in planned educational efforts. The hospital stay is more likely to proceed smoothly when there is effective communication among professional staff and when the advice and information offered to the mother is consistent. Nurses should be clear when offering advice that it is only advice. The mother should feel free to disregard it if she should so choose. Mothers valued moral support from staff because this initial post-partum period is a profoundly emotional time. They appreciated it when staff expressed a personal interest and when they communicated warmth and understanding. Simple words of encouragement and small acts of kindness can have a marked impact on the mother's confidence and can go a long way toward starting her off on the right foot. When women encountered difficulties they often attributed them to the busyness on the ward and a shortage of time. Often mothers had to take the initiative. They had to seek the information or ask for help. Unfortunately, such initiatives could require too much effort on the mother's part in those early post-partum days. When problems arose, and nurses were pushed to capacity, the system broke down: 'When I did have problems, then the system really broke down. It was really a question of me going to them and basically saying, "Can't somebody please help me?" And they really didn't do a hell of a job. They've just got too many assigned duties that have to fit into the prescribed schedules and that's it.'

At certain times it is inevitable that staff on maternity wards will be extremely busy. Often this will be the time when problems arise. It is therefore imperative that formal policies and procedures be instituted that support the breast-feeding mother so that the impact of these constraints is minimized.

Hospital policies are frequently singled out as an important target for changes that would improve breast-feeding rates. Kitzinger (1979) has noted, however, that 'most hospitals are ill adapted to fostering the subtle and important relationship which is developing between mother and baby' (p. 72). Position papers published by the Canadian Paediatric Society (1978) and the Canadian Home Economics Association (1979) recommend implementation of policies to enhance women's experience of breast feeding. Many Canadian hospitals are now adopting such policies but the problem is often more with the day-to-day implementation than with the intent. Ongoing staff training and monitoring will be necessary to avoid the types of communication problems experienced by the women in this study. Four studies of post-partum care in Alberta hospitals found similar problems and reinforce the need for continuing vigilance to ensure that hospitals respond flexibly to the needs of mothers and babies (Harvey and Post 1986; Field 1985; Filshie, Williams, Osbourn, Seniour, Symonds, and Baskeit 1981; Houston and Field 1988).

CHAPTER SIXTEEN

Physicians

Doctors may influence women's experience of breast feeding because of their repeated contact with them during pregnancy and the early months post-partum. If physicians encouraged preparation in the pre-natal period and offered support and practical advice post-birth, breast feeding could be easier and more rewarding. Physicians, however, must be careful how they interact with mothers because they are seen as authorities on infant and child care. Their remarks can have a strong impact on women's behaviour and self-esteem. Women who feel unsure about their ability to master the tasks of mothering are vulnerable; even well-meaning advice can be misinterpreted and lead to problems.

Support from the Doctor

Because the women we interviewed had differing interpretations of what constituted support there was a wide range of physician behaviour that was considered supportive of breast feeding.

Doctors who placed pamphlets on breast feeding in their waiting-rooms or stated their preference for breast feeding were described as supportive by a few. However, the bulk of the comments characterized supportive behaviour as active physician involvement with the mother and her baby. This included supplying information on breast feeding and infant health, allowing time to listen to and talk with the mothers, and giving the mother feedback on the baby's progress.

Doctors were viewed as an important source of information and advice. Women turned to them for help in such things as understanding why the baby had gas or colic, or was crying. They often wanted to know what range of behaviours was normal and, therefore, questioned doctors on the baby's bowel movement and frequency of crying or feeding. They questioned whether they should breast feed when they had yeast infections, whether their diets affected the baby's bowel movement, how to treat painful breasts without decreasing their milk supply, and how to continue to breast feed after returning to work. These women were dissatisfied when practical advice was sought but not received. Some discovered that their doctors had limited knowledge on the management of breast feeding and on how to cope with the vicissitudes of a new baby. They questioned their doctors' credibility when information or advice ran contrary to what they had learned from their own experience.

Women wanted the opportunity to talk to their doctors. They needed sufficient time to ask questions, to voice their concerns, and to talk through their problems. They hoped for a sensitive and empathetic response. Unfortunately, women frequently complained they had too little time with their doctors. They felt rushed and left the appointment with their problems unresolved. The manner in which mothers were sometimes treated in these brief appointments compounded their negative feelings. Although Fern trusted her doctor's judgment, she was frustrated when her problems were not addressed. The light atmosphere that was maintained was not conducive to getting down to business. She recalled: 'I was a little put off by him. You go in there with such a long list of complaints and he ends up talking, joking, and laughing about something else so you forget what you were in there for in the first place. When you get home you think, "Gee, I didn't get to talk about how miserable I feel."'

Mary was another mother who spoke at length about the lack of time with her doctor. Mary's baby had colic and she felt desperate in the first few months after his birth. She labelled her physician's practice as assembly-line medicine, a term that captured the quick, mechanical nature of the visits. She recalled some of the difficulties she had had:

I didn't feel like I could talk to the doctor about things. The problem was sort of getting dismissed. We didn't think the baby was getting enough to eat. The doctor said, 'He's getting plenty to eat.' I thought he was very fussy. The doctor said, 'Just give him this stuff' and that was it. There was no time to discuss things. He had these printed forms done up and he'd circle what you had to do. It was quite obvious he really didn't want to get into the ins and outs. He had three rooms going. You talk about assembly-line medicine. The nurse would set the kids up and he'd come in and give the needles. He was very pleasant and very nice but you just didn't feel like you were getting the support.

For Mary, support meant having a doctor care about not only the baby but also the mother. She expected the doctor to be sensitive to her concerns. She elaborated on her expectations:

I felt that I needed support. I felt I should have gotten it from the doctor. Even if he listened a bit more it would have been nice or if he'd given a couple more ideas on what to do. One thing I found a help was putting a hot water bottle under Marty's tummy. These sorts of things. The doctors don't care about these little bits and pieces of things. It doesn't seem to make that much difference to them whether you were up all night or three nights on the trot, get no sleep, and that sort of thing. It should be important to them. The attitude more or less is that caring for a baby is easy. You've been foolish about this, but this will all be over in a little while and all that sort of stuff.

Time with the doctor was equated with having an attentive, understanding, caring listener with whom to talk. Mary found that the doctor's involvement could not be assumed and that, in her instance, an 'arm's length' relationship was more likely to be maintained: 'I got nothing from professionals in any way. They're at arm's length, not involved in the particular situation. They don't take time to find out. You go to a doctor and you start to tell them what it's about and instead of encouraging you to talk and explain the situation, you're handed a prescription; and if you try to go into it in any further, well, that's going to take care of it.'

Mary and other women like her wanted moral support from their physicians. They resented being shuffled in and out of doctor's offices without being given enough time to voice their concerns. They wanted understanding and empathy. Again Mary summarized for other women when she said: 'Go to a doctor that listens to you. You don't want to have to explain everything. But you want a doctor to ask you questions. You don't want to feel that you're moaning and all that sort of stuff, though I think you have a right to moan.'

Most of the women interviewed were the principal caregivers, at least during the first few months, and were strongly focused on the growth and development of the baby. They felt responsible if the baby was not developing at the expected rate. Because it was the doctor's role to monitor the infant's development their comments were taken seriously. Doctors who expressed confidence in the physiological mechanisms of breast feeding reinforced mothers' confidence that breast milk would adequately nourish their babies. Because many women associated their ability to breast feed with their capacity to be good mothers, the doctor's reassurance was particularly important. The impact that the doctor could have was summarized by Pamela: 'I feel that it's really important to have this discussion with the paediatrician about his or her beliefs related to breast feeding because it will make a big difference. Those appointments are very important for you. All you have to hear is that baby's not getting enough to eat and I'm sure then you're going to feel totally responsible.' Another woman remarked how a 'wrong word can just devastate you.'

Women expected to be reassured that their baby was developing normally. Because mothers could see for themselves whether the baby was healthy they could usually anticipate the doctor's comments. None the less, mothers talked about needing the doctor's reassurance that their assessment was correct. As Lisa remarked, 'I knew what he'd say, but I just wanted to hear him say it.'

Many physicians not only provided reassurance but also praised mothers for the fine job they were doing. When Charlotte went to see her doctor and the baby weighed in at 11 pounds, 6 ounces, Charlotte was delighted to be told, 'Whatever you're doing, you're doing well.' Her next appointment was delayed because of the baby's excellent progress. Feedback like this bolstered self-confidence.

Other physicians offered practical advice that supported breast feeding. For instance, Ellen recalled: 'My doctor was in today and said the important thing about breast feeding is to make sure you get enough rest. He said, "Sometimes you're feeling really great and think you're doing fine but if you don't get enough rest then it can affect the milk," which is very true.'

Halina's doctor appreciated that nursing served more than a nourishing function. After her baby was given a needle her doctor suggested she retire to his office to nurse because the baby could use the comfort.

Some women were disappointed to discover that physicians they had identified as pro—breast feeding were not as supportive as they had hoped. Knowledge of physiological mechanisms that govern milk production, the adequacy of breast milk, and the role of other influencing factors seemed to be lacking. Some physicians blamed breast milk for difficulties that arose with the baby and suggested the introduction of a formula supplement. Mothers confronted with these recommendations reacted with feelings that ranged from indifference to devastation. The following examples illustrate the impact doctors had when they suggested a supplement as a solution to difficulties or concerns. Marian had identified her paediatrician as someone who was 'all for breast feeding; he never pushed solids.' Later she discovered that most of the women she met at the doctor's office were not nursing. Marian worried that her doctor would recommend a bottle if she complained about the baby's fussiness or if the baby was not gaining weight as expected. The potential impact of the doctor's remarks is evident in Marian's readiness to deceive him to avoid upset:

Well, the paediatrician didn't really help. I never said, 'You know, I think she's hungry.' He probably would have said, 'Give her the bottle.' In fact, I had already decided that. I could see she'd gained weight by the time we went for the first visit. But I had decided that if she looked little to me a week before the first visit I was gonna give her formula. Because I knew that if she wasn't gaining he would say, 'Stop breast feeding. Give her the bottle,' and I didn't want that. So I had decided that I wasn't even gonna tell him that there was a problem 'cause I knew he wouldn't support breast feeding.

Pamela described her son as a big healthy baby, 'a little giant' of 11 pounds at eight weeks. When she went in to see the doctor, she mentioned that she was feeding frequently because the baby was so hungry. She recalled the conversation with her doctor:

He said he could understand that by looking at his growth rate, which has been quite rapid since birth. He said, 'Yes, he is hungry, so of course, he is requiring more feedings.' And, of course, once again his answer was to supplement. That would give him what he needed and would also give me relief. And so I said, 'Well, I hadn't supplemented as he'd said. I had given maybe, all in all 8, 10, 12 ounces in the last month.' But he said, 'Give him as much as he wants every day, at one feeding, even up to 10 ounces,' which just about floored me because I've been giving him one ounce or two ounces and thinking I had given him quite a bit.

Pamela was unaffected by her doctor's suggestion. She

believed that he was trying to decrease the burden on her and was not questioning the worth of breast feeding. A woman with less self-assurance might have taken the doctor's suggestion as a criticism of her ability to nurse, followed his advice, and weaned the baby off the breast. Jennifer was one such woman.

Before her son was born, Jennifer had asked her doctor about his views on breast feeding. She recalled that 'he seemed quite positive about it.' Then she heard after the birth that the baby was not gaining enough weight. She panicked and wondered if she had enough milk. Her doctor's attitude at that time was, 'he'll survive both ways, with breast milk or formula.' Jennifer understood this to be a suggestion to supplement. She subsequently weaned the baby. Later Jennifer wished she had continued nursing. She wondered, in retrospect, if it had been necessary to introduce a bottle at all because her baby cried after the bottle just as he had done after nursing. She concluded that the doctor had unwittingly started a chain of reactions that eventually led to weaning: 'I wasn't sure if he was saying that just to make me feel okay. I don't think he said it as a deterrent to nursing. I think it was more that he wanted me to feel, "Well, your child's going to be okay whether he's nursed or not."'

Jennifer's doctor appeared sensitive to the fact that she might not consider formula to be as good as breast milk and tried to quell her concerns. He probably did not recognize that Jennifer might feel a sense of failure if she did not breast feed. Jennifer linked breast feeding to her sense of self-worth: 'When I nursed him and he cried in between or during, I kept thinking I'm doing something wrong. But when he just takes a bottle and he cries, well, it's not as personal an attack.'

Sometimes recommendations to supplement resulted in a stronger desire to succeed at breast feeding. Fiona and Laurie (whose case studies appear in chapter 6) were both told that their babies had not gained enough weight because of inadequate breast milk and that they should supplement with formula. Both women were devastated by their physicians' comments. Fiona talked about feeling 'like a very incompetent female, guilty as a mother, with all kinds of negative feelings.' Laurie said she felt 'stupid and inept and guilty.' Both of these women believed that breast feeding was part of being a good mother. To fail at breast feeding was to fail at motherhood.

Fiona and Laurie were determined to continue breast feeding whether or not they received encouragement from their physicians. Fiona turned to La Leche and Laurie to books to learn how to avoid giving up breast feeding. Both pumped their breasts and discovered they had plenty of milk. They then were able to dismiss their doctors' attribution that they had insufficient milk. Nevertheless both women paid an unnecessary psychological toll as a consequence of their physicians' feedback.

The Doctor/Mother Relationship

Many of the difficulties described above may have had their roots in the type of relationship that existed between the mother and her doctor. When the doctor was seen as or acted omnipotent, mothers were placed in a subordinate position and were less able to interact in an adult fashion. When the relationship was viewed as collaborative or advisory, women were less likely to feel deficient in their abilities to manage problematic situations.

The 'doctor as authority' was considered an expert on infant feeding because he or she presumably had years of training and experience in handling babies. Physicians in this role dictated appropriate behaviour, such as what to feed the baby and when. It was assumed that the mother would trust the doctor's judgment and would follow advice even when it ran contrary to her own instincts or to other advice she had received.

A few women, who saw doctors who had an authoritarian attitude, were content with the relationship that developed. Fern, for example, talked about trusting her paediatrician's judgment without question. She speculated that her ease with this type of relationship arose from her training. She had worked as a nurse and was accustomed to taking orders from doctors. She felt very close to her paediatrician.

Nadine also looked to her doctor as the expert on child care. She did not see herself as the person who should make certain decisions about her child. She explained that she was not accustomed to doing things on her own. Nadine talked about taking cues from her doctor. For example, she gave the baby pablum and banana only after the doctor recommended that they be started. Nadine responded to her problems by relying on the doctor's opinion. When the baby was thought to be anaemic, Nadine remarked: 'The doctor didn't seem too worried so I didn't get really neurotic about it.'

She trusted her physician and simply accepted his judgment. She felt guilty when she acted without checking with him first. When her baby was sick, and she breast fed him, she questioned whether she had done the right thing: 'I don't know if the doctor knows that I'm still breast feeding. He said not to give him any formula or anything. And with some guilt, I did give him a nibble from the breast.' Nadine's guilt suggests there is an element of paternalism in the doctor/mother relationship. Nadine believed her conduct should be regulated by her doctor's opinion and she felt badly when she acted without permission.

A number of women felt trapped in a childlike role with their physicians. Elizabeth thought her physician acted like a 'dog trainer,' who spoke to parents in a very 'condescending' manner as if they were 'stupid.' Elizabeth believed her doctor would judge her negatively if she did something 'wrong.' She therefore avoided creating situations that would cast her in the role of 'bad girl.' For instance: 'The other day the paediatrician said, "Oh, you've lost too much weight. You're losing your breasts." I didn't say that I didn't care if I had them or not. She'd probably think that I didn't want to be a mother.'

Patsy, too, was unhappy with both doctors she saw: 'My doctors were both pains in the neck. I had very poor relationships. I had two different doctors. I changed after my first because I really felt uncomfortable with him. He treated me like I was some little girl, like, "How dare I ask the great big doctor any questions about my pregnancy?"' Patsy was also irritated because she had expected her doctor to be an authority on and advocate of breast feeding but found she had to rely on her own resources to prepare for nursing. Patsy recalled one of her visits to the doctor: 'I said to the doctor, "Do you encourage breast feeding?" He looked at me as if I had two heads. It's almost like they don't care. They don't give you any advice on how to prepare your breasts. If I hadn't been reading my books, I would have done nothing to prepare the nipples.'

Physicians themselves may believe they are simply offering (as opposed to dictating) advice. However, if they adopt an air of authority they risk structuring a situation in which women feel that there is only *one* right way to proceed and that their own expertise or viewpoints are discounted. Mary's comments capture the thoughts of a number of mothers in our study:

When you're with professionals you always get the feeling there's a right and wrong, no in-betweens. If you don't do what they tell you to do you're being a bad mother. You're setting the doctor up for problems and you're into all kinds of guilt feelings.

It's almost as if they take away the choice, your instinct. You feel that you can't go with your instinct because you're told this is wrong and that's wrong and you should be doing this and you should be doing that.

Mary did not deny her doctor's expertise: 'You know I tried to go along with what the doctor said. He's had all these babies; he knows what he's talking about. You've only had one or two. It's been a long time and you've forgotten a lot of things. You don't really think that this is going to work but you should try it because he knows. He's the professional.' The problem arose because the advice did not work. There was no mechanism for joint problem solving, so Mary turned totally to her own experience and instincts to guide her: 'It was only when I started completely disregarding what he said and went with what was working – that's when things worked out. Now I go with what I feel. We're not doing things according to the book.'

Some women were not troubled by their doctors' authoritarian stance. They simply followed the advice when they agreed with it and disregarded it when they did not. One of the women we interviewed was Bess, a physician herself. When Bess's doctor learned how frequently she was nursing he suggested introducing formula. Bess commented: 'I've been resisting that. I told him how I felt. He didn't listen. So I went ahead and did what I wanted to do.' Although Bess was not willing to follow his advice, it was important to her that her doctor not think she was ignoring his recommendations. As a physician, Bess was interested in her own response: 'I'm really getting insight into non-compliance. Not only am I not doing what he says but I'm sufficiently convinced that if he continues to make an issue of it [trying formula], I will start lying to him. 'Cause I like him as a doctor in other ways and I don't want to trash up our relationship. But if he insists, and cannot accept my way of doing things, then I'll just start lying to him. And so I'm beginning to see this side of it [patient's point of view].'

The doctor in the role of colleague was someone who collaborated with the mother in choosing what should be done with the baby. Both the doctor and mother assumed that the mother was able to weigh information and come to decisions on her own or that she might wish to share the decision making with the doctor. It was important to mothers that their opinions and ideas be valued. These women did not like being judged or dismissed when they reacted to what the doctor had to say or when they expressed their concerns. Furthermore, they did not want to be pressured. As one woman pointed out, 'Doctors do have a way of swaying you into doing things' and this pressure was unacceptable to women who wanted to participate in decision making. Halina's comments illustrate shared decision making: 'I have a very good paediatrician. I really have a lot of confidence in what he says. He's a type of guy who stands back and says "Let's see what happens." With the baby's staph infection, instead of dictating he said, "We could either give her some cortisone cream or we'll just leave it." I'd prefer to leave it.' The doctor suggested two approaches and provided the opportunity for Halina to choose either option.

Daisey also found a physician with whom she could establish a collegial relationship: 'She seems to be very easy to talk to. She certainly didn't say anything negative about what I wanted. She didn't say, "I'm the doctor so whatever I want, you're going to have."'

A collegial relationship was satisfying because women's opinions were valued and because they could participate in decision making. Dissatisfaction with a physician's role usually arose because of a lack of fit between the mother's and doctor's expectations. Women who did not want an authority relationship thought such doctors were rigid and unaccommodating. Nevertheless, many established a working relationship by listening to the advice and then acting as they saw best. In a collegial relationship, because decisions were made jointly, the atmosphere of compromise, flexibility, and shared responsibility meant that women were not placed in a position of having to ignore advice and worry about the consequences.

Specialist Confusion

Of the women interviewed, a small group complained that lack of support arose because physicians were not available after the birth of the baby. They felt deserted and forced to find other support persons or resources on their own.

Cheryl was one of the mothers who felt this isolation. Her comments were as follows: 'I don't know who you are supposed to call when you are having a problem nursing. The paediatrician or the obstetrician ... both sort of wash their hands and say that's your own problem.' Cheryl eventually discovered that the La Leche League was her best source of help.

Violet also commented on the lack of support in the post-partum period. She said: 'The doctor didn't give me any assistance at all. During the pregnancy she didn't really take any interest in my breasts or how they were. It surprised me that you really are very much on your own. It's up to you to read the books and to find a network or someone that you could turn to. Afterwards when he was a few months old, I didn't know whether it was the paediatrician's area or the obstetrician's area. Everybody left you to your own devices.'

Violet was not alone in feeling confused about which specialist to turn to. Women wondered who was responsible for helping them manage their breasts for breast feeding. Christina shared some of the confusion she felt: 'It's funny with breast feeding because who do you ask? I asked my obstetrician a couple of things, but she's an obstetrician and a gynecologist, and the baby's doctor, who's a paediatrician, is interested in the baby, not me. I could have gone to my GP, but I don't like him that much. I really didn't know who I should ask about my breasts.'

Earlier studies have found that many mothers viewed their physician as unhelpful with regard to breast feeding (Martin 1978; Sachs, Brada, and Hill 1976; Sloper, McKean, and Baum 1975). A more recent study indicates a shift in attitude among physicians (Lawrence 1982). It concluded that they recognized the importance of increased professional and educational support. However, there was evidence of role confusion among the sub-specialties about whose role it was to support breast feeding, and a substantial minority of physicians believed nothing should be done to encourage longer breast feeding.

One recent development is the emergence of professional lactation consultants who are certified by the International Lactation Consultant Association, of which there is a Canadian affiliate. To qualify, individuals must have completed a bachelor's degree, continuing education related to breast feeding, and 2500 hours of lactation consulting, and must pass an exam. Although there are currently just over 100 certified consultants in Canada, their numbers are expected to increase. They provide specialized support for nursing mothers, particularly those in crisis. Although many consultants are self-employed, some are now working in positions in public health, hospitals, and clinics.

There is a basic set of knowledge and skills that doctors can acquire to help them support the breast-feeding mother. First, doctors need to acquire an understanding of what the experience of breast feeding is like. They need to appreciate the emotional nature of the experience, the inherent isolation, and the accompanying fatigue. To understand the difficulties that arise, doctors must appreciate that breast feeding requires skills and is not just an instinctual response. They need to know what those skills are, how to teach them, and how to deal with the difficulties that do crop up. Second, doctors need to appreciate the relationship between self-esteem and breast feeding. The confidence and self-esteem of some women will be precarious and easily undermined. This problem demands that doctors learn to give feedback in a sensitive, supportive manner and to recognize the potential impact of their comments on women's self-confidence. Finally, physicians need to appreciate that all mothers are individuals with unique experiences, difficulties, beliefs, and values. Individual differences need to be acknowledged and respected to enhance each woman's experience of breast feeding.

Doctors have an elevated status and visibility among other health professionals and the public. They are assumed to be knowledgeable on most matters dealing with the functioning of the body, including breast feeding. These assumptions may explain why some women preferred lying to challenging their physicians' expertise and why some would discount their own common sense in deference to a physician, who may have no actual experience with breast feeding or child care. Some of the problems described in this chapter might be resolved if women could transform their view of the physician from that of an expert to be obeyed to that of an adviser who is prepared to help with problems. This role transformation cannot take place in isolation. It must be accompanied by a shift in the way in which physicians view and act on their roles. It may also require the provision of more non-medical support services such as telephone hot-lines, drop-in centres, and support networks similar to the La Leche League.

CHAPTER SEVENTEEN

Family Relationships

Breast feeding occurs most often within the family milieu. Ideally, it should be the place where a woman gets the most support for her role as a breast-feeding mother. In reality, this was not always the case. In many instances husbands or partners were preoccupied with employment concerns and left the parenting and home-making tasks to their wives. The changes that accompanied a new baby led to new stresses in the marital relationship. Other family members, particularly parents and in-laws, grew up at a time when bottle feeding was the norm. They were not impressed by breast feeding and sometimes actively discouraged it.

In contrast, there were examples of positive family support. These examples are helpful in building images of the kinds of support that all women deserve as they bear and nurture children.

Husbands/Partners

Almost two-thirds of the women interviewed discussed their husbands/partners. The comments ranged from brief notations of their husbands' opinions of breast feeding to long discussions on their husbands' involvement (or lack of) in parenting. Four aspects of parental relationships will be described. These include husbands' attitudes towards and support for breast feeding, how the relationship between mother and father changed with the arrival of the baby, the role that husbands played in housework and child care, and, finally, the nature of the couple's sexual relationship after the arrival of the baby.

Attitudes and Support

Somewhat surprisingly, most women in this study had little to say about how their husbands or partners supported their efforts to breast feed. A few made general comments about the importance of husband's bringing the baby to be nursed, occasionally diapering the baby, and helping by taking on some of the household chores to ease the pressure on the mother's time. The bottom line, in terms of support, was partner involvement, not only by helping with the household tasks but also by expressing interest and concern about the details of the mother's preoccupation with the baby and other family matters.

Most women believed their husbands wholeheartedly approved of nursing. Husbands' views on the superiority of breast feeding appeared similar to those of their wives:

When I first started to breast feed, I was surrounded by some negative people. My husband was very positive. My husband never expected me to do anything else. My husband was sure we were having natural childbirth and breast feeding and that's what happened. I think he got offended when people seemed negative about breast feeding.

I think he would have been very upset if I hadn't breast fed. I think he would have thought that I was doing my child an injustice. He was more pro than anything.

Breast feeding absorbed large amounts of time and energy and decreased time available for household tasks. Because of the frequency and timing of the feedings, it often happened that every time the husband saw his wife, she was nursing: 'He'd leave in the morning. I'd be nursing. He'd come home at night. I'd be nursing. And maybe during the day, you'd nurse all day and you'd be frazzled in that.'

The husband's response to this could be crucial. In the following example the husband's lack of sensitivity created problems:

The first month mostly we were just about to separate. It was terrible. He didn't understand. He didn't expect me to go through this depression for such a long time and to such an extent. I was constantly breast feeding, and I mean constantly. Every time she cried I was in her bedroom nursing. I didn't take her out of the house. I didn't vacuum. I didn't do all the housework type things. He used to come home and say, 'What did you do all day?' 'Well, I breast fed.' He said, 'Is that all you did?' And so forth. Every time he criticized me I started crying and I wouldn't talk to him and it was like a chain reaction. He didn't want to say anything because he was afraid to offend me. And it was the cold war, no conversation. Eventually I breast fed less and less. I had the juices and I left her with him when I went out a few times and things were getting a little better.

A more supportive attitude was appreciated. Dinah said of her husband: 'I couldn't have done it without him; he's terrific. He believes in it 100 per cent and wouldn't want it any other way. And at my hardest times, he just pushed me.'

In a few cases the husband played an active role in influencing how long his wife breast fed. Hannah's and Tracey's husbands were both influential in prolonging breast feeding when their wives wanted to give it up. Hannah continued breast feeding at her husband's request: 'I must admit that I wanted to quit breast feeding before I did and my husband kept me going. He kept begging me to stay, to keep her going, that it's very good for her and he would really love it if I could keep her on it. If it wasn't for him I would have quit before.'

Tracey's husband reminded her that breast milk was the 'best thing' for the baby: 'It was lucky I have a husband who was really encouraging breast feeding because at times when I was getting really uptight and upset about it, I would say I'm giving up and he kept saying, "But Tracey, you know it's the best thing for him."'

One woman felt pressured by her husband's desire to see her continue breast feeding. Kim's husband, a physician, was strongly in favour of breast feeding and constantly pointed out the benefits to her. She described his persistence and her conflict:

I felt like Brian really wanted me to breast feed. He really did not want me to bottle feed. A large part of it was the financial reasons. He kept saying, 'Gee, that's another $10 on our budget for the week.' I felt I was really trying to stick with it just to please him. Through the time that I'm breast feeding he seems to come up with all the material in his journals on how it benefits the baby and gives them to me. I'm reading this stuff and there in the back of my mind somebody's telling me, 'No, it's time to stop.' I'm not really happy with it and at the same time he's really pushing it on.

Kim's husband's enthusiasm for breast feeding blinded him to Kim's need to have some relief from nursing. Kim believed her husband did not really understand the difficulties she was experiencing: 'What's hard is that he's not home all that time that I'm going through this. I think he has to actually be in my shoes for that 24 hours and he'd think differently.' Kim would have preferred the type of support that Agnes's husband offered: 'He would have supported me either way. He never suggested, "Oh, she's not getting enough, give her a bottle." But at the same time, when there were times I said, "Oh, God, I can't stand this, I'm gonna wean her," he'd say, "Well, if you want me to give her a bottle once a day" to sort of try to accommodate me.'

Some women were concerned that the father might feel excluded from developing a close, nurturing relationship with the baby because he could not do the feeding. Melanie spoke about this:

Any sensation I might have had about his being left out probably came from me and my concern. I was always aware that that can happen to new fathers and I'd say, 'Do you feel left out? Do you wish you could do this?' Or, 'Come and be with us, and sit with us, and talk with us while I'm feeding Mark.' It didn't seem to bother him too much, and especially now that Mark is starting to respond to him. He's very playful. I think Lance doesn't feel as left out anymore. He can feed Mark his cereal. So he's now beginning to contribute to that part of Mark's growing up.

Fathers who became involved by bringing the baby to the mother to nurse, and who burped, changed, and bathed their infants, had an opportunity to develop a more intimate relationship. This helped the nursing mother and she was also rewarded by seeing the relationship develop between father and child.

At the other extreme, Estelle and Cheryl were certain that their husbands supported breast feeding because they did not want to be bothered feeding the baby. Estelle said: 'He's been delighted that he hasn't been able to actively feed them. He thinks it's marvellous that he can sleep through the night and not feel guilty. Because he can't feed them anyway. He thinks that's the biggest advantage of breast feeding as far as any father should be concerned.' Cheryl believed the same thing: 'I think he always wants me to breast feed so that he doesn't have to feed the baby in the middle of the night. He doesn't like me to do it for the bonding or anything. I'm sure he likes me to do it so that he doesn't have to feed.'

Changes in the Parents' Relationship

The arrival of the baby and the attendant changes in life-style could have a major impact on the relationship between the nursing woman and her husband. As Jennifer said: 'It's culture shock for both of us. It's still trying to fit in that we're not just two people anymore. We're two people who have a little child who's dependent on both of us.'

Women who discussed the impact of a baby on the marital relationship most often focused on the negative aspects:

Having a child is very disruptive to a relationship. We have both found that. There are definite rewards but also some drawbacks. One is trying to establish the relationship as it was before. I don't think you can ever do that. You have to make allowances for change and find a happy medium. That's work!

My husband was going through a rough period with his job too. So it's a period of adjustment for all of us. Our marriage went poof. Right down. We're having just a tough time.

One of the more common sources of difficulty was the shifting of the woman's attention from her husband to her baby. Iris spoke about this aspect:

When he'd come home from work and wanted to tell me about his day, he didn't have my undivided attention and couldn't always get it. Sometimes he'd say to the baby, 'Hush, it's my turn!' He found it hard to adapt, to really accept it. I couldn't just ignore whatever the baby was doing at the time, especially if I was nursing him. You have half your mind on them all the time anyway. So no matter what your conversation is, if baby makes a funny noise, you're distracted. I think he found that hard.

Sherri also talked about not having time for her husband: 'It was a little rough at the beginning because of the neglected husband type of thing. It felt like there was no time for him anymore and really when you're nursing and when you're taking care of a baby all the time, you do tend to forget about him for a while. It was a bit rough on him at the beginning.'

Fatigue and lack of time curtailed the amount of interaction between a woman and her husband. There was often no time to simply sit and talk. The time when the husband came home in the evening was often the baby's fussy period and the mother was occupied with that. Later on, she was too tired to stay up with her husband. In some cases, because of the isolation, her husband was a woman's primary link with the outside world. She depended on him to satisfy a need for adult interaction. Knowing that her husband would come home at the end of the day helped her to get through. This dependence could place an additional strain on the relationship. A woman might also vent her frustration on her husband at the end of the day. Sonja described this: 'It's the adult conversation and the company and somebody that's the same size as you are. I think you hold it all in and slug them instead of the kids.'

While a negative change in the marital relationship was not an inevitable outcome of a new baby, it appeared that women spoke primarily about those situations that were distressing. The following quotation illustrates a situation where a relationship benefited from the arrival of the baby. The mother explained: 'It's just enhanced because we feel a different joy in our relationship. We look at our child, we feel a different joy. We laugh and we say we're tired, but we're not interested in doing those other things any more either. Even if we weren't tired, we're not particularly interested in going to see the latest show.'

The management of housework strained some relationships. Because of the baby, less time was available to do the usual tasks and new arrangements had to be worked out. This posed difficulties for Lisa and her husband: 'Our marriage has really been tottering the last few months. That's one major problem. It's mainly because he's not taking on full responsibility for being a father.'

In the situations where the husbands were unwilling to share, problems often arose. A typical example is illustrated in the following excerpts from an interview with Terri: 'It was Labour Day and we were home all day. Jason was sleeping for part of the day and Pete was looking after him for the other part of the day. I was rushing around madly trying to get the cleaning done. And Pete said, "Why can't you even relax when I'm home?" Well, it was the only time I could do something. He doesn't seem to understand that.'

Terri believed that her husband should have known that she needed help: 'I just feel like he should realize that I don't have to ask him to do something. He should realize that he could help. So, I don't know if it's pride or what, I don't bother to ask. I do it myself and I'm a real martyr about it.'

Part of the problem arose from the fact that the arrival of the baby had altered the way Terri and her husband split tasks: 'When I was working, Pete and I split our household chores. The expectation was when I quit work, housework was my job. Except I don't know if Pete realizes how very tired I am at the end of the day and I would really like some help with dinner. So, I just go about and do everything and I think, "Well, fine, OK! You watch your TV and I'll do it. I'll be a martyr and I'll let you know in my little ways."'

Fern noted the importance of good communication, especially when fatigue compounds already complex situations: 'My husband and I had a big flare up on Saturday about the division of duties. I felt he wasn't doing enough. I spent an hour in tears. Maybe we need to do a little more of that. He's tired, I'm tired. We're vulnerable to disagreement. He's being helpful. There's just times when he doesn't snap the way I think he should. My husband says we are trying our best. He says if I have genuine concerns I should let him know and he will try to improve.'

Husband's Role at Home

The husband's involvement in the household management and child care ranged from almost nil to heavily involved. Most women said their husbands shared at least some of the housework. Often women qualified the amount of their husband's participation by explaining that he did as much as he could given the time available after work. Darlene said: 'He's trying to help as much as he can. He's been great, cleaning up and stuff every night. He's insisted on getting all the dishes done and out of the way. He's really busy with work, too. So we're both doing as much as we can.'

Other women described how their husbands participated. Lisa, for instance, described her husband as 'very good': 'He pitches right in there with the diapers and the bottle feeding and on weekends he alternates with me just about everything. He feels regret that he doesn't have more time during the week. Weekends are really the only time for him. And he feels badly about that.'

Hannah's husband assumed more responsibility as they had more children: 'My husband helps very much. If he's home in the day, if he's working at night, he will cook for me when I get home. Or he would wash the clothes. He's very helpful. He helps more and more as I have more kids. He just took on more responsibility.'

Agnes described how her husband altered his work schedule so that he would be home in the evenings to help her out: 'Matt really shared the whole thing, very much so. He came home from work and that was it. He was fully involved and normally he would have to go out in the evening and do estimates for his job and stuff, but he just did them all either on the weekend or squeezed them in during the day. So once he walked in the door, if he had left, I would have killed him. I mean I desperately needed him. If he hadn't been here, I would have been a wreck.'

Pamela's husband took over a large part of the housework, which allowed her to give her baby 'the kind of time he seems to require':

I'm so caught up in giving 100 per cent of my time to Aaron. When I've seen how much Will has done for us to allow us that kind of time together, I have to really give him a lot of credit for that kind of support. He'll have a very nice supper on the table, a very nutritious supper after he's been at work all day. He does a lot of looking after Aaron, too, all the time. He wants to be a part of everything. As far as those other tasks are concerned, like the laundry, and dinners on the table, and grocery shopping. I haven't done any of that. Not that I'm saying it has to be definitely the woman's role to do that, but I used to share those responsibilities.

Pamela's husband seemed to have the most enlightened view of father's sharing described in this study. In many cases, the father's contribution to housework and child care had distinct limits. He rarely had to put up with the daily difficulties that are part and parcel of baby care. There were frequently qualifiers that explained these limits. The following comments were common in the interviews:

He gets frustrated. He really doesn't have the same amount of patience I do.

He doesn't like changing diapers now. He tries to get out of it. They smell since the baby switched to formula.

I definitely do more for her than he does. I tend to think of her as my job. He looks after her when I go out.

I don't find him as helpful as he was with my first. He's taking a night course. He usually helps around 7 with one of the kids but then he starts studying.

I can't blame him. He's not the type to do baby care. He's scared of little babies. He wouldn't do anything until she was about a year old.

My husband usually has time with my daughter in the early morning. But lately he's been leaving home very early because he's joined a club. He works out in the morning and plays squash.

With his new job being so busy he's either out or he's sitting at the dining room table working like mad. He's not the type of person that delves right in with children because he's had no experience with children.

He likes to hold her when she's quiet. If she's crying it gets him upset.

He doesn't know what to do. He seems to like holding her as long as she doesn't throw up on him.

Women tempered their expectations of their husbands because they knew their partners would be tired at the end of a day's work. A few women, whose husbands had either started new jobs or were having a particularly busy period at work, were totally responsible for housework and child-care. Marla and Jennifer both accepted their situations without complaint:

He's so busy with his work that he's not here that much. It's not really bothering me because with his job being so new, I feel that he's going through a pretty rough time. So I don't mind taking whatever burdens I can off him. I know that they don't really have the division of roles in society that they used to have and yet I don't mind having that.

He started a new accounting course, which is taking up a lot of time. And he was promoted at work, so there's been so much happening within the last three weeks that with Bill I try not to be too demanding because I don't think it's fair. I'm starting to realize he does work all day and when he comes home at 9:30, if he's working late, he's tired, too, and I don't like to lay a trip on him.

Other women found their husbands' long and stressful work days more difficult to accept. Bess, a physician who took a year off between medical school and interning, recalled her reaction when her husband worked late for three weeks. He would come home at midnight, and leave again the following morning at seven. She described the conflict that arose:

He's my major social contact and I need him. Also I feel that the baby needs him and sometimes I feel that he doesn't realize that. I said, 'What if I'm interning and this happens?' He said, 'Oh well, we'll get a baby-sitter for her.' What did we have her for? Let's send her back to the hospital or throw her out? I felt pretty badly about that, but his boss has just quit and he's applying for his job so he'll have better hours. I figure I've quit my job for a couple of years. He can do it, too. He doesn't feel the necessity of it. I just sometimes feel that if I don't do the parenting nobody will. That's not exactly the kind of situation that is easy for me to then go into an internship. I may be wrong. I'm probably overreacting. What can you do? You can lead a horse to water but you can't make him drink it. Sometimes I'd like to shake him.

In time these tensions were resolved, largely because of how Bess's husband's work evolved.

Mary coped with a colicky baby all day. Her husband was experiencing a lot of work-related stress. At the end of each day both partners felt the need for empathy and support. Unfortunately, neither had their needs met: 'Thomas was having a rough time. So when he came home he didn't have time, inclination, or anything else to be really supportive. He was looking to me for support and I was looking to him for support and neither of us would give any support anyway. It's only been in the last while that it's improved and then, of course, I went back to work and I found that really difficult.'

Kim described how difficult it was to cope by herself all day and throughout the evening:

He wasn't home when I really needed him. That was the hard part. Like at 11 at night he'd really try to motivate me to breast feed but he wasn't there when I really needed it. Most husbands will come home at 5 or 6 at night and I *needed* that. I just needed to say, 'Take them, I wanna go out for a walk or I wanna do this, or talk about my day.' I didn't have that. He would come in at 11. I would be pacing up and down with him screaming. He'd come in the door and I would just shove Simon to him. I would say, 'Take him, I can't handle it any more.'

It helped Kim to know that her husband understood how demanding mothering and housework were: 'He really understands, that's one good thing. He really is supportive and he understands how I feel. He doesn't know how I do it, how I stay at home with two kids all day. He'll do it sometimes on a Saturday and he's ready for the mental hospital by the end of the day.'

Similarly, Marla said that it was her husband's acknowledgment of how much she did that kept her from resenting the lack of help from him, especially since he was under a lot of pressure in his new job: 'He knows how much I do. He realizes and he mentions it: "I know you're being very good and I thank you for being understanding." He lets me know that he knows and that's fine with me. If he didn't and I felt that I was being taken advantage of, I would be upset.'

A few women noted that even though their husbands were helpful and tried to be understanding, they did not have a *true* understanding of how stressful and demanding looking after a baby on a daily basis could be. Lorna and Fiona commented: 'As much as my husband does understand, in some ways he doesn't understand the stress of just being with a baby all day.' / 'My husband, he's a super guy, in terms of what he's done, in terms of his role with the baby. He's done more than any husband I've seen. But yet, as hard as he tries to understand me, and he really tries sincerely, he still doesn't really appreciate the fact that I have two jobs.'

Many women were undemanding of their husbands and were willing to subjugate their own needs in deference to them. Perhaps they thought their husbands' needs had greater value because they were linked to employment and income. Husbands and wives were both exhausted at the end of a day, yet many women were reluctant to make demands because they believed their husbands needed their rest. Women carried on alone with meal preparation and child care despite their own exhaustion. The preferential valuing of paid employment, which reflects the values of our larger society, must be questioned when its consequence is the devaluation of women's work in the home.

Some husbands did share responsibility for household chores and child care. Many, however, participated only occasionally. They 'helped out,' which is different from sharing the responsibility. These situations reflect traditional sex-role norms in which men are not expected to participate equally in work in the home. When the father's employment and other activities occupied an excessive amount of time outside the home, he abdicated his parenting responsibilities to his partner.

Sexuality

About one-quarter of the women talked about sexuality in the first six months post-partum. Most said that sexual interaction with their partner was slow to resume once the baby arrived because they were too tired or too emotionally absorbed with the baby. Most women assumed their lack of interest was temporary and were not particularly worried about their feelings.

Although the majority of husbands accepted the situation, a few had difficulty. Dinah described why she was not interested in sex and how her husband felt about it:

Definitely he feels replaced and we still have that problem because first of all breast feeding has affected me sexually. I don't have any desire and on top of that is the fact that she doesn't sleep very much. I don't have very much rest. All my emotion goes into her, and I have very little time left for him that way. He's my best friend and I couldn't do without him, but from my side, I'm satisfied. Emotionally I'm satisfied with her and on the other hand, except that he's more tired, nothing has changed for him. He has all the desires he had before and he doesn't have a wife anymore. That's been really hard on him. It's been hard on him and hard on me because I feel so bad for him because I'm so torn between him and myself and her, trying to please three people at once and nobody gets satisfied, especially me.

Dinah felt that the relationship she had with her husband before they had the baby was gone and expressed regret at its passing: 'We weren't married very long before she was born and we had a wonderful, wonderful relationship and we both kind of feel sad that it's gone. We are still the best of friends, but I mean in terms of how intimate we were able to be before.'

She also believed their relationship had become unequal: her husband was giving to her but was not getting anything back because she was emotionally drained by the baby: 'Any need to give I give to her, unfortunately. All my giving is to her. She demands it. I don't have any choice. I would like to share it, but she doesn't give me that chance. Whereas any getting I need, which isn't much these day, comes from my husband. My husband is giving but he is not getting love, so in that sense it's harder on him. He's feeling bereft. But then I suffer in other ways. I feel bereft of sleep.'

Other women also talked about reduced sexual activity because of their own lack of desire. Low sexual drive was common during pregnancy and over the period that women breast fed. Sometimes, if a woman had had two closely spaced children and had breast fed them both, sexual relations with her partner were affected for a long period. Sybil and Kay described their situations:

Your relationship sexually with your husband is altered temporarily. And also just your relationship with him because you're so preoccupied with the baby. You don't have the same amount of time and ability to do things together. It's not spontaneous. You have to plan things now. But if you both genuinely wanted the child and feel good about that you put up with a lot in the short term because you know it's not going to be forever. The sexual relationship, just because of having a child, is affected, regardless of whether you're breast feeding, just because you're feeling uncomfortable down there. I think initially your fatigue is just so overwhelming that you have absolutely no desire at all. I had a desire to be held close, and to feel that closeness with Greg, which I do, and that's fine, but actual sexual feelings I don't think were there.

The worst thing that I find with breast feeding is I have very little sexual satisfaction. Not sexual satisfaction as much as sexual feelings. I feel very, very loving, but, and it's the same when I'm pregnant, I have no desire whatsoever for sex. It does make a long stretch of time, especially with two kids. The other thing is, you always wonder if it's ever going to come back.

Maintaining open communication is an important part of coping with these changes. Robyn and her husband both had a diminished sex drive and Robyn described how they approached this issue: 'As long as we talk about it and we're open about it and try to do something about it. I force myself. I'll put on something a little bit sexy and try and see. Sometimes I will, and my husband is too tired. It's funny. We just have a good laugh sometimes about it and we try to see what we can do. We're quite open about it. It was a shock finding I didn't want to make love but it's coming back now – slowly but it's getting there.'

A few women described a loss of sensitivity to sexual stimulation in their breasts and also of feeling uncomfortable about their breasts being touched in a sexual way while they were still breast feeding. Gillian talked about her lack of response:

One other thing about breast feeding is that I am so used to her sucking that I don't have a lot of sensation that a woman would have sexually. I think once I've stopped, it will go back, but in terms of arousement and things like that, I'm so used to someone being there all the time, that it's not as easily stimulated. Because it's happening six times a day, when it comes to having a sexual encounter it's not a big deal – who cares, I mean it's nothing. But I think that will change once I've stopped. It doesn't bother me.

A few women were concerned that their breasts would leak when fondled. It was this fear rather than a feeling that the breasts were for the baby that made them hesitate to have their breasts touched:

I didn't have the feeling that it doesn't belong to him. I was more concerned about the milk coming in – like I didn't want all of a sudden to be sprayed in the face or dripping. That, I think, makes you a little more self-conscious when you're with your mate. You're thinking, 'Oh God, I hope my milk doesn't come out right now.'

In some situations it's not all that enjoyable. For example, if you are making love with your husband and your nipples start leaking you have this milk all over the place. It certainly puts a damper on everything. It's difficult enough as it is in the beginning. Here they are, leaking right in the middle of the whole deal. It's not too appealing, especially since my husband is a very neat person. It sort of throws him off.

A couple of women talked about sex being painful because of a decrease in vaginal secretions. One woman believed this was a factor women should take into consideration when making the decision to nurse:

When sex starts to hurt you, it just makes matters worse. Thank goodness it's not half as bad as I anticipated. For a lot of women it is. And they're just not prepared for that. Couples should know. I think when women are making the decision to nurse at the very beginning, that's an important variable. To us, sex is important along with the rest of the marriage. But there are some people I know to whom it's an everyday important. And if these people are looking at nursing they should really know.

Unlike most women, Susan found that although she was ready for sexual interaction with her partner, he was avoiding it: 'The first, maybe four months, Mark almost avoided me. I was up on a pedestal, the new mother. I would say to him, "I'm no different, I really need to make love." But we didn't. It was a nasty time. He still avoids my breasts. Like it's almost like it's a bit sacred. And for that reason sometimes I think I've just had enough of breast feeding.'

Orissa's husband also had difficulty with her dual roles of mother and sexual partner:

A couple of days ago he said, 'Well, don't you think that six months is a long time to breast feed?' I said, 'It seems that she still has the need to breast feed and it doesn't bother me at all. It really doesn't put a strain on me in any way.' The only thing is that it limits me publicly. It's not enough to stop me from breast feeding. My husband says, 'You're wearing all those ugly bras all the time' and 'here you are with the milk supply so it's hard for me to relate to you sexually because it's hard to differentiate the mother.' It's almost like the madonna – the mother figure. How can you perceive a mother figure also as a lover? It's difficult for him to see the two together. I said, 'Well, what do you want to do? Do you want me to buy those tiny bitty bras which never fit?' He said, 'Get some nice looking bras. You don't have to wear those horrible things.' So we haven't resolved this conflict yet because it's more comfortable and more convenient for me to wear those bras you can just undo. She takes priority. So it's not sexy, definitely not sexy. But that's his problem.

Sometimes, the decreased interest in sex is mutual, with strong parental instincts replacing sexual drive. Daisey described the changed feelings toward sex that she and her husband had:

Both my husband and I feel very much like our sexual feelings have completely disappeared. We don't even have any sense of it at all. Our whole world is around the child and the paternal and maternal feelings are so strong. I think that's really nice, to feel that when you have a child you can forget about those sort of feelings. We both feel that our feelings toward sex have changed dramatically. For me, personally, my whole outlook on life and everything seems to have changed with motherhood. Also, my husband expressed some change as well. Not just in the basic things like responsibility, but his feelings toward me. The feelings sexually are downplayed a lot because the maternal and paternal instincts become so strong. One tends to think of sex almost on the spiritual level more so than it ever was before. That it's a creative thing rather than a physical gratification.

A few women reported having satisfactory sexual experiences. Melanie described her situation:

As far as sex with Lance goes, or just the relationship with him, I haven't found it to be inhibiting to him at all. I was worried initially that I was very leaky and messy and that I wouldn't be appealing. I also felt just kind of blobby and droopy. That was the general self-image I had, with the extra weight I was carrying at first. But I think he kind of enjoys the fact that breasts are more than just appendages, you know, stimulating appendages. I think he likes the fact that they serve a function and that they can make him happy and make Mark happy. It's that dual purpose. He's kind of an efficient person, maybe that appeals to him. They're not just hanging there for no reason at all.

Cynthia said of her sexual relations: 'It gets better and better. He sleeps through the night and goes to bed around nine so we've got our evening. The odd time we take advantage of the afternoon, if he's sleeping. We have to be flexible and realize that's OK. It's not a night-time-only type thing, especially on weekends. If he's having an afternoon sleep – terrific!'

Fern and her husband knew from their experience with their first child that it took time to recapture their interest in sex. It took a year and a half to get back to normal. Fern commented: 'When it does happen again and you are both ready. It's nice to feel you can still appreciate it. But it does take a long time.' Fern also described the importance of her husband's attitude towards her body:

I am fortunate that my husband is very patient and loves me very much. So my body isn't what it used to be! He says I'm still beautiful to him even though I moan and groan about my body, that I can't manage to get it into any sort of shape. I have a couple of friends whose husbands are sarcastic about their appearance. That would crush me if my husband felt that way about me – if he didn't want to touch me. He loves the way I look and enjoys my body the way it is. We manage to maintain a special closeness.

Other Family Members

After husbands, a woman's own mother and mother-in-law were the family members most frequently discussed. They could be either a benefit or a hindrance to the nursing mother. Those who were described as supportive were sensitive to and respected the new mother's decision to breast feed even though they may not have breast fed their own children. They did not interfere or offer unsolicited advice. They visited shortly after the birth and helped out by cooking, cleaning, and caring for the mother. Ginny's mother was typical of these women: 'I just didn't feel I had to be a mother all the time. My mother was looking out for me. Mothers don't care about grandchildren, husbands, or anybody as much as they care about their own child. That just made me feel a little bit better. Just having her here was nice.'

The women we interviewed spoke more frequently about parents and in-laws who were not supportive. They were seen as interfering if they expressed scepticism about breast feeding. Their lack of support could be subtle or blatant. A simple glance from one's mother could be devastating to a woman who lacked confidence. Examples of such undermining behaviours include:

I had never realized how strong an influence my mother had on me. In general she hasn't, but I was insecure enough that every time she would look at me with that worried look on her face I would be ready to run for the bottle. But I kept at it through pure stubbornness.

My mother wasn't supportive at all. My sister wasn't supportive. They made it seem like it was something that was not really filthy but, you know, not a proper thing to do. Unclean in some way, I guess. Unsanitary in some way. How could you give the breast to the baby? You should be giving them sterilized nipples and bottles. I said, 'Well, I'm going to do it for six months.' Six months approached. My mother would say, 'Well, it's six months. She's too old already to be breast fed.'

My mother-in-law made me feel like I was participating in an act of pornography or something. When I was suffering from the pain and the soreness she said, 'Why do you go through with it? My three children grew up perfectly well and weren't breast fed.'

My mother called and of course she's got all kinds of advice. Now she's completely turned off breast feeding because everything has not been going well. She's just sick to think it's because Aaron's starving. This is her grandson – and I'm starving him. She's talked to a lot of women. She hasn't had one positive experience expressed to her from her generation or my generation. She wrote me a very nice long, concerned letter and talked to me on the telephone. So by Sunday night I was really beginning to feel that probably I should just switch over to formula.

You can imagine the advice I was receiving from my parents, 'No wonder the baby is cranky. Your milk isn't good enough. It's not thick enough. He's quite obviously starving.' I kept saying, 'No, he hasn't had a bowel movement, I'm sure that's the problem' ... 'Well, of course, because you don't give him water.' 'But you don't have to.' I say, 'because breast milk has enough water' ... 'Well, there you are. You see, it's not rich enough' ... It's awful, just awful.

Nursing mothers expended valuable energy fending off these types of comments expressed by well-meaning mothers and mothers-in-law.

Sisters and sisters-in-law were the only other family members who were mentioned frequently. Those who had children usually served as role models and supplied both emotional support and practical advice to the nursing mother. A few, however, like those parents described above, undermined the nursing-mother's confidence in breast feeding with their unthinking comments.

The transition to parenting brings about many changes in marital relationships. Some of the changes are transient but many will be more permanent, at least until the last child has passed through infancy. As the primary care-giver, the mother is focused on the needs of the new baby. There are very real constraints on her time and she is less able to attend to the needs of her husband. Conflicts over roles and the sharing of responsibilities frequently emerge. The conflicts are often exacerbated because former levels of intimacy have been fractured by changes in the sexual relationship and coping with fatigue. It is a time when extra care must be taken to ensure that communication channels stay open. Both partners need to be sensitive to the other's point of view. It is often impossible for men to empathize with their partners' experiences because they cannot imagine the work of mothering. It is difficult to articulate the panoply of mixed emotions this role generates. There is great joy and tenderness, overwhelming fatigue, laughter, anger, frustration, pride, loneliness, confusion, and love. These are all superimposed on a role that demands thirty-five-hour days. Relationships will be enhanced when fathers begin to share the role more equally and learn, first hand, what it means to 'mother.'

Other extended family members can be supportive by offering to help with household tasks, to baby-sit, and to listen with empathy. It is important not to criticize the mother's behaviour or attitudes. She needs support for her efforts and should be given advice only it if is requested.

CHAPTER EIGHTEEN

Other Sources of Support

There were other important sources of support aside from family members and health professionals. These included friends, support groups, and books. These were more significant when the mother did not have sufficient support from her immediate family.

Friends

Friends who had children, and particularly those who had breast fed, were able to share experiences and offer advice and reassurance. Interactions such as the following were welcomed:

Friends phone me up and they'll ask how things are going. If you ask them a certain question they'll always come back with, 'Oh, yeah, that's what mine did.' It always helps. Everybody's been giving advice or personal experience.

It is important to have friends that are at the same stage as you are. They're more willing to listen and I'm more willing to listen. We're wanting reassurance and we do some comparing and we keep saying we have to keep this in perspective.

I had one good friend who's breast feeding. My baby was born two weeks after hers and she was the greatest source of support. She went through the exact same things and it made me feel like I was normal and not something out of the ordinary. It really eased the anxiety of loneliness. I felt so alone because there was no one physically around me. I was supported just over the phone.

A few women were disillusioned with the support they got from friends. Some believed their friends were less than frank about what breast feeding was really like. Betty, for example, claimed that women 'smooth things over. They just say they have bad moments but it's worth it in the long run.' Betty felt cheated. She wished somebody had 'sat down and said, "Idealistic views are nice but these are the cold cruel facts."' She went on to say: 'I sat there in a fog before I had a baby. People told me this stuff but they didn't use the right words like "devastating." Things were said, like, "It's pretty hard." What's hard? The worst I'd ever felt before this was a severe hangover. This has got it beat by miles. That's all I had to relate to as far as feeling bad.'

Support Groups

Support groups were an ideal place to get information and reassurance and many women sought them out. The groups ranged from the La Leche League to those organized by community centres, churches, health units, YWCA groups, and sometimes by the women themselves. Mothers used the time at these groups to share experiences and enjoy each other's company. Some groups offered a number of services including baby-sitting, play facilities for children, and speakers on a variety of topics of interest to mothers. Most of the women gave glowing reports of these groups. The only complaints focused on subtle pressure to conform to a group standard defining what they should be doing as mothers. This was particularly so in the case of the La Leche League but this weakness was balanced by many other strengths. Because the La Leche League was the group most frequently mentioned and because women had strong feelings about it, both pro and con, it will be discussed in more detail.

La Leche League

The La Leche League is an international support group for women interested in breast feeding. Local leaders, who have breast-feeding experience, conduct meetings in their own homes so breast-feeding women and those who want to learn more about nursing can meet to gather information and support each other. League leaders are also usually available by telephone at other times if additional support is needed.

Many women were extremely satisfied with the La Leche League. Practical advice offered by league members worked. Wisdom shared from league mothers' experiences was accompanied by information known to be 'backed up medically' and was seen to be 'not just hen-party type information.' Because many mothers doubted health professionals' knowledge of breast feeding they relied heavily on the La Leche League: 'They're really the people who are the experts. I think what they say is correct. I think most health professionals really do not know enough about breast feeding.'

Many women used La Leche to confirm their doctor's recommendations: 'The doctor prescribed antibiotics. I just wasn't sure what it would do to the breast feeding. So I called the La Leche League. She said, "There's no problem." That made me feel a bit better. Hearing the doctor say it didn't reassure me as much as hearing one of La Leche League people. I know the doctor is right and I did believe her but it was also reassuring to hear it from the La Leche people.'

La Leche leaders offered important moral support. They provided encouragement and reassurance that mothers were doing well in their breast-feeding efforts. This support and empathy gave a boost to many women. Pamela, for instance, said that the La Leche leader in her area 'made me feel good. The things she was saying I totally believed in.' Pamela went on to say: 'They were very supportive of my concern. They didn't necessarily give me any advice that I hadn't thought of or I hadn't read about but they were supportive when I needed some advice. I felt I could phone them. There is a real need to have support when you're embarking on something you know nothing about.' Pamela and other mothers appreciated the accessibility of La Leche women – they were as close as the telephone, twenty-four hours a day. Even if they were not used, the knowledge that they were available was sufficient support for some women.

There were a number of women who expressed reservations about the La Leche League. The most common concern was the traditional view of motherhood that is part of La Leche philosophy. If this was pushed, it could create resistance. Estelle believed that league members 'tend to come on much too strong.' She explained: 'There's a lot of things the league stands for that I agree with, and yet when I have a league member talking to me about it, I feel like my back's against the wall and I wanna come out fighting. Yet, it's things I believe in.'

A few women compared the approach taken by some league members to that used by religious fanatics. When league members were dogmatic they were labelled as patronizing, inflexible, and overbearing. In response, women felt belittled and guilty. This was particularly true of women who requested information on weaning choices upon returning to work or the decision to introduce a formula supplement. Tracey had called La Leche for advice because she wanted to wean her baby. She was upset when she was told her baby was too young at three months. Tracy concluded that La Leche was 'too pro–breast feeding for somebody who's not able to breast feed or makes the choice not to.'

La Leche has a long history of providing support for women who breast feed. For many years, when breast feeding was not popular, it was one of the few available sources of support. It was on the leading edge of the groups advocating a return to breast feeding. Today it continues to provide advice and emotional support for countless women. The sharing of practical wisdom founded on the experiences of women who have breast fed is the hallmark of this group. However, certain members express such strong opinions about the superiority of both breast feeding and traditional roles for mothers that some women become upset with the advice offered. Others would avoid calling because they anticipated a response that would not meet their particular needs.

Books

Books were another source of support. First-time mothers read avidly both before and after the birth of the baby. Women expected books to provide them with the knowledge necessary to breast feed successfully. They liked books that had common sense, were down to earth, and affirmed their experiences with breast feeding. Books also reminded women that their difficulties were not unique, an important function when women were isolated from one another: 'I remember looking on *The Complete Book of Breast Feeding* almost as the Bible in the hospital. I would find things that I was experiencing in this book. It was just great to know, hey, it's not just me. I'm not just the weird one and something's wrong. This is a perfectly normal thing. To mothers the first time around, I think something like that is very helpful.'

Books bolstered women's confidence: 'It was very encouraging in terms of helping me really believe that my milk was what the baby needed and that I shouldn't be blaming my milk for different problems. It helped me realize that people in the past had done that by saying that you needed to supplement, that you didn't have enough milk or had too much milk. My milk wasn't to blame!'

Some women believed that books had not prepared them adequately for what was to come. From reading, they had developed an image of breast feeding that did not fit their experience. For example, the baby fed and was awake more frequently than the books had suggested, or the baby's weight increased at a rate different from the book's charts, or the baby did not eat the amounts prescribed. It was noted that most books did not mention that breast feeding might not work. This omission made the decision to discontinue breast feeding before the recommended time more difficult for some women.

Mothers were shocked to discover how sore and exhausted they were; they were not alerted to the emotional impact of mothering nor were they prepared for the emotional drain on their energy and ability to concentrate. They were confused by the dissonance between expectations and experience. Books were blamed for some of the resulting turmoil. Christina, for example, concluded that 'all the books are full of shit.' Margaret believed the books created unrealistic expectations: 'When you read in a book that a baby's supposed to feed every four hours and sleep twenty it's kind of damaging. That sets your expectations. Not many mothers have that good a chance of attaining that.'

Some women found it difficult to identify with what they were reading before the baby was born. They read about the joys and difficulties of breast feeding but the scenarios portrayed remained outside of their experience. They were not perceived as the 'real thing.' Intellectually they were prepared; emotionally they were not: 'On an intellectual level, all the researching and reading on both breast feeding and delivery is very helpful. But on an emotional level, it's basically useless. You can read and read. You have an understanding but it's too text-booky. It's just not completely real.' When the baby arrived the emotional response came as a surprise. One mother said, 'Even though I'm intelligent, I'm emotionally upset.' Another noted, 'You get emotionally uptight. You don't think properly.'

Support, throughout this emotional time period, is extremely important. A variety of approaches to providing support need to be considered. Clearly, books such as this one, that present a realistic picture of breast feeding, are needed. There should be easy access to support groups. As well, neighbourhoods need to be designed to promote interaction by providing facilities including parks and local community centres where mothers and children can meet.

PART SIX

Conclusion

CHAPTER NINETEEN

Promoting Breast Feeding

To study the significance of breast feeding for women it is necessary to examine it as part of the broader process of having a baby and to understand the nature of the sociocultural context in which this entire experience takes place (Maclean 1989b). In this way we can develop a more integrated understanding of the interplay of personal and environmental factors that influence women's experience and of the steps that can be taken to enhance breast feeding. In particular, it is important to note the societal barriers that spring from attitudes towards women's roles, sexuality, mothering, and the importance of children. It is unusual for health professionals to pay attention to such issues but a minority of writers are stressing the need to fully integrate issues related to women's reproductive activities into the *public* life of society (Arango 1984; Helsing and King 1982; Van Esterik and Greiner 1981).

We can see from the material presented in this book that breast feeding is a complex activity that is intimately tied to a woman's sense of herself. Women's approach to breast feeding and how long they continue to do it are influenced by a wide range of factors. Some are psychological factors related to the attitudes, values, and character traits of the mother, the baby, and those close to them. Others can be labelled structural factors and encompass such things as the absence or presence of formal and informal support systems that cover the range from paid maternity leave, community drop-in centres, and educational programs to community parks where mothers can meet. There are also a host of cultural factors that influence the way nursing mothers and those around them view breast feeding. These would include socially mediated norms around ideal body shapes and weight, women's breasts, and women's and men's roles.

There is a vast professional literature on the psycho-social influences on breast feeding. However, this study is one of a very small number of studies that have examined breast feeding from a holistic perspective. Of these select studies, this one is the most comprehensive in terms of sample size and range of issues examined. The findings, particularly those that reinforce the multitude of complex factors influencing women's experience of breast feeding, are confirmed by published reviews that synthesize the literature on this topic. The most recent of these, by Kearney (1988), supports the significance and interdependence of the psychological, structural, and cultural factors that influence breast feeding.

The range of individual responses to breast feeding in the study was as broad as the range of influencing factors. Some women loved it and breezed through. Others hated it. They were disappointed with what happened. Breast feeding did not bring that special closeness to the infant, and mothers were frequently exhausted. At first they felt excruciating nipple pain when initiating feeding. Later they leaked 'like cows.' It was virtually impossible to find a moment of free time for themselves. There were other women in the middle range, who at times felt great tenderness and warmth while breast feeding but at other times felt burdened and depleted. For these women ambivalence was part of breast feeding but they recognized that it was also part of being a mother.

Breast feeding cannot be isolated from the larger experience of having a baby. The addition of a new family member heralds a whole set of changes for the mother and within this context breast feeding also brings changes. Indeed, the concept of change or transition has been increasingly used as a thematic focus to examine what happens to couples and families following the birth of a baby (La Rossa and La Rossa 1981; Miller and Sollie 1980; Oakely 1979, 1980). It is change – in responsibilities and use of time, in women's bodies, and in personal needs – that helps explain the meaning of breast feeding in women's lives. It is through an examination of the potential impact of these changes that we can identify the strategies that can be used to encourage and improve women's experience of breast feeding.

Changes in Responsibilities and Use of Time

The first few months post-partum are very demanding on a woman's time. The mother is the primary care-taker of the baby and any older siblings. Because she is nursing she is solely responsible for the feeding activity. For many mothers the early months are characterized by frequent feedings and unpredictable feeding schedules. Night-time feedings mean interrupted sleep patterns and extreme fatigue. A mother can spend up to twelve hours a day nursing during the first six to twelve weeks of the baby's life.

As a result of these time demands women have little or no time to meet personal needs, to relax with their husbands, or to pursue social or recreational activities. Because the baby's behaviour and needs are unpredictable it is virtually impossible to make firm plans to do anything. Women often feel totally disorganized. Even if they find some free time they might be unable to make effective use of it simply because they are too exhausted to do anything but sleep.

Women, particularly first-time mothers, must learn to accept that life with a new-born is demanding and to recognize that their usual standards related to daily accomplishments are inappropriate during this period. It is important for a mother to take a relaxed attitude to housework and meals and to use any time left over after child care to pamper herself.

Many young women today are accustomed to being in control of their lives. They are organized, efficient, and used to taking the initiative and seeing things fall neatly into place. It is a shock when they realize they are at the mercy of an infant. It can be disorienting to discover that one can no longer accomplish even the more mundane tasks of daily life.

In our culture the definition of effective use of time is derived from the business environment. Time is viewed as a commodity that is to be controlled and managed with the aim of increasing productivity. Successful time management is rewarded by increasing levels of accomplishment, which are usually measurable. This particular orientation towards time is inappropriate when it is applied to the tasks of mothering. Because babies' behaviour can rarely be controlled, mothers are usually in a position of responding rather than actively managing. Coupled with fatigue, the day-to-day activities of baby care can leave almost no time for anything else. Child-care activities are frequently intangible. At the end of any given day a mother might look back and conclude that she has 'accomplished' very little. A societal emphasis (often implicit rather than explicit) on observable achievement subtly undermines the importance of many of the less tangible mothering tasks. Many mothers in the study bemoaned their lack of daily achievements, at times implying that they were verging on slovenliness. There was also an implied belief that the activities of child care were not work in the same sense that paid employment, which their husbands did, was work. Many women were reluctant to make demands of their husbands, particularly at night, because they had to 'work' the next day. Although these women knew their brief day-time naps would be unlikely to compensate for their lack of sleep, it was apparently more important that the husband be the less fatigued of the couple, presumably because of the value attached to activities that receive financial remuneration. By comparison, the responsibilities of mothering are seen as less important.

It is essential that both the nature and the value of women's work in child care be re-examined. It may not be necessary to place a dollar value on the work but it is important that its merit be recognized and that it not be devalued in comparison with work that receives direct financial remuneration. It is also important that the work of child care not be divided totally on the basis of gender. Although breast feeding will remain the responsibility of women there are many other tasks that can be shared. More enlightened policies such as paternity leave, job sharing, and flexible work schedules are needed to enhance the perceived social significance of parenting and to facilitate a more equal sharing of parental responsibilities.

Recognition of the effect of the baby's temperament on breast feeding is an important factor in adjusting to the changes. It was clear from our interviews that babies, like everyone else, display a range of temperaments, and women who understood that fact were less likely to attribute problems to breast feeding. As well, babies displayed very different feeding behaviours. Some wanted to feed every hour and a half whereas others wanted to feed every three or four hours. Some maintained regular intervals between feedings; others did not. Some babies started sleeping through the night at six weeks of age; others were not sleeping through at six months. These differences simply reflected the differing personalities of the babies. Mothers with other children often commented on the differences between their children and feeding behaviours were no exception.

Body Changes

There are substantial changes in a woman's body during pregnancy and in the weeks and months following delivery. Many women gain enough weight during pregnancy that it will take a number of months to lose it after the baby is born. Few of the women we spoke with were complacent about the extra weight. They complained about the size of their hips, waist, and stomach, and worried about stretch marks. Leaking breasts were an irritant to many women because of the mess, the inconvenience, and their emotional reaction to them. The most significant impact of these body changes was psychological. Some women hated the new shape of their body and referred to it with disgust. They claimed they could not feel good unless their appearance was to their liking. The frequent use of the word 'cow' conveys the sense of the distaste that some women felt for their body and its maternal functions. A few women who had gained excess weight with their first pregnancy found it so distasteful that they were prepared to breast feed only briefly so they could get down to the serious business of dieting.

Weight control and body shapes are an obsession in our society. As women we have been socialized from an early age to believe that thin is beautiful. Boyish figues are in; maternal figures (with the exception of large breasts) are out. We have spent much of our lives being critical of our bodies. At the time when women's bodies are the farthest from the so-called norms, it is difficult to tune out our own critical voices and accept what has happened to our bodies as a normal outgrowth of maternity.

At the same time that women are struggling to accept their bodies as they are, they are discovering, if they venture to breast feed publicly, that there is a social antipathy to their bodies as well. At a time when women's breasts are freely displayed on the front pages of local newspapers it is unacceptable to discreetly expose one's breast to feed an infant. It is more acceptable to feed in toilets than in public places.

These social influences and their manifestations are often subtle and many women may be quite unaware of their impact. It is little wonder that these influences create ambivalence and confusion during a period that is already fraught with powerful emotions. It is inappropriate to blame individual women for being irrational about their bodies. Instead we need to look at the social determinants of these attitudes and seek ways to reorient them.

Changes in Personal Needs

The addition of one new, completely dependent family member increases a woman's responsibilities substantially. Women with new babies have increased needs for physical support in the home with child care and household management. First-time mothers, in particular, need knowledge about the physiology, techniques, and problems related to breast feeding and infant care. All women need emotional support and recognition and valuing of the mothering role and of their efforts to breast feed. Breast feeding in this study was unanimously viewed as superior to bottle feeding and many women wanted their unique contribution to the baby's welfare recognized. As well, many women craved temporary relief from the responsibilites of mothering and breast feeding so they could have some time for themselves.

The need for information on breast feeding is crucial. There are many excellent books available about the techniques of breast feeding but few of these prepare women for the emotional responses to breast feeding. Although reading before birth can be helpful, it is sometimes difficult to absorb the information until you are actually faced with the situation. It is, important, therefore, that women have access to information in the hospital when they are initiating breast feeding. Pamphlets, video-tapes, and formal teaching are all needed. Once the mother goes home she needs continuing access to information. Once again books are useful. But women also need the opportunity to discuss difficulties with a knowledgeable person so they can make informed and thoughtful decisions about how to proceed. Although women in the study group looked to physicians for this type of support, many were too busy or unwilling to provide it. Health professionals could benefit from educational opportunities that would teach them more about the support needs of new mothers who are seeking advice. Some women found La Leche helpful but others avoided it because of its sometimes dogmatic position on women's roles. Some found other groups that met their needs, but there was clearly a gap in support services. Too many women were unable to find support when they needed it most. Health professionals, pre-natal organizations, and women's groups need to work together to publicize their services and to develop creative ways to fill the gaps.

Family structure, income, housing, and neighbourhood also influence women's needs. Women who live in extended families or who have family support nearby are more likely to get physical and emotional assistance. Women who live in neighbourhoods where there are young families often share baby-sitting and give support to each other. Neighbourhood parks play an important support role. Women can join friends in the park, but, more significantly, the park provides a place to meet new people and thereby lessen the isolation many women feel.

From the study we know that women living on lower incomes face additional problems. They are more likely to live in apartment buildings and feel isolated from their neighbours. There is less money for baby-sitting. They are less likely to have a car and, therefore, have to rely on public transportation to get out with the baby. There is a need for financial support for local community groups to develop strategies to support women in these situations. Funding can be used to develop parent/child centres, to organize baby-sitting cooperatives, to develop a lending library of books and toys, or to develop networks of mothers who are willing to lend a hand to one another.

As the emphasis on women's roles has shifted to the issues of enabling women to contribute equally in the work-force there has been less acknowledgment of the important contribution women make in bearing and raising children. Women are placed in the position of having to remind themselves of the value of their nurturing work and having to seek recognition from those who share the same experience. It is important that women's groups direct their attention to improving the situation of all women who have children, including those who choose to stay at home. It is a disservice to all women to dichotomize women's roles and to ignore the issues that fall within the realm of reproduction and family life.

Many recommendations directed towards the promotion of breast feeding have focused on changes that women as individuals can make to improve the quality of their experience. They stress the need for educational programs that provide the necessary knowledge base for successful breast feeding. However, as the findings from this study illustrate, there are many factors that influence the course of breast feeding that are beyond the control of individual mothers. Contextual factors play an important role in breast feeding. These include the structural realities that are manifested in concrete barriers to breast feeding and the more subtle socialization processes that influence a woman's response to her own experience. All concerned individuals must work together to press for changes in our socio-cultural environment so it will be easier for women and men to nurture societies' children.

References

Adair, L. 1983. Feeding babies: Mother's decisions in an urban U.S. setting. *Medical Anthropology* 7: 1–19

Allen, L., and G. Pelto. 1985. Research on determinants of breast feeding duration. *Medical Anthropology* 9: 97–105

Arango, J. 1984. Promoting breast feeding: A national perspective. *Public Health Reports* 99: 559–65

Auerbach, K., and E. Guss. 1984. Maternal employment and breast feeding. A study of 567 women's experiences. *American Journal of Diseases of Children* 138: 958–60

Bentovim, A. 1976. Shame and other anxieties associated with breast feeding: Systems theory and psychodynamic approach. *Ciba Foundation Symposium* 45: 159–78

Bogdan, R., and S. Taylor. 1975. *Introduction to Qualitative Research Methods: A Phenomenolgical Approach to the Social Sciences.* New York: John Wiley & Sons

Bogdan, R.C., and S. K. Bikien. 1982. *Qualitative Research for Education: An Introduction to Theory and Methods.* Boston: Allyn and Bacon

Brack, D. 1975. Social forces, feminism, and breast feeding. *Nursing Outlook* 23: 556–61

Cable, T., and M. Rothenberger. 1984. Breast feeding behavioral patterns among La Leche League mothers: A descriptive survey. *Pediatrics* 73: 830–5

Canadian Home Economics Association. 1979. Infant and child feeding position paper. *Canadian Journal of Home Economics* 29: 199–201

Canadian Paediatric Society. 1978. Breast feeding: What is left besides the poetry? *Canadian Journal of Public Health* 69: 13–20

– 1979. Infant feeding. *Canadian Journal of Public Health* 70: 376–85

Carlson, S. 1976. The irreality of postpartum: Observations on the subjective experience. *Journal of Obstetric, Gynecologic, and Neonatal Nursing*, 5: 28–30

Chapman, J., M. Macey, M. Keegan, P. Borum, and S. Bennett. 1985. Concerns of breast feeding mothers from birth to 4 months. *Nursing Research* 34: 374–7

Clarke, S., and R. Harmon. 1983. Infant initiated weaning from the breast in the first year. *Early Human Development* 8: 151–6

Cronenwett, L., and R. Reinhardt. 1987. Support and breast feeding: A review. *Birth* 14: 199–203

Feinstein, J., J. Berkelhamer, M. Gruszka, C. Wong, and A. Carey. 1986. Factors related to early termination of breast-feeding in an urban population. *Pediatrics* 78: 210–15

Field, P. 1985. Parents' reactions to maternity care. *Midwifery* 1: 37–46

Fieldhouse, P. 1982. Behavioral aspects of the decision to breast-feed. *Canadian Home Economics Journal* 32: 88–97

Filshie, S., J. Williams, M. Osbourn, O. Seniour, E. Symonds, and E. Baskett. 1981. Post-natal care in hospital – time for change. *International Journal of Nursing Studies* 18: 89–95

Florack, E., G. Overmann-De Boer, M. Van Kampen-Donker, J. Van Wingen, and C. Kromhout, 1984. Breast-feeding, bottle-feeding and related factors. *Acta Paediatrica Scandinavica* 73: 789–95

Giorgi, A. 1970. *Psychology as a Human Science*. New York: Harper & Row

Glaser, B., and A. Strauss. 1967. *The Discovery of Grounded Theory: Strategies for Qualitative Research*. Chicago: Aldine Publishing Co.

Graef, P., K. McGhee, J. Rozycki, D. Fescina-Jones, J. Clark, J. Thompson, and D. Brooten. 1988. Postpartum concerns of breastfeeding mothers. *Journal of Nurse-Midwifery* 33: 62–6

Grassley, J., and K. Davis. 1978. Common concerns of mothers who breastfeed. *American Journal of Maternal Child Nursing* 3: 347–51
Greiner, T., P. Van Esterik, and M. Latham. 1981. The insufficient milk syndrome: An alternative explanation. *Medical Anthropology* 5: 233–47
Gruis, M. 1977. Beyond maternity: Postpartum concerns of mothers. *American Journal of Maternal-Child Nursing* 2: 182–8
Gunn, T. 1984. The incidence of breast feeding and reasons for weaning. *New Zealand Medical Journal* 97: 360–3
Gussler, J., and L. Briesemeister. 1980. The insufficient milk syndrome: A biocultural explanation. *Medical Anthropology* 4: 145–74
Harrison, M., J. Morse, and M. Prowse. 1985. Successful breast feeding: The mother's dilemma. *Journal of Advanced Nursing* 10: 261–9
Harvey, L., and S. Post. 1986. Changing patterns in maternity care. *Canadian Nursing* 15: 28–34
Health and Welfare Canada. 1982. *National Survey of Infant Feeding Patterns: A Synopsis*
Helsing, E., and S. King. 1982. *Breast-feeding in Practice: A Manual for Health Workers*. Oxford: Oxford University Press
Hewat, R., and D. Ellis. 1984. Breastfeeding as a maternal-child team effort: Women's perceptions. *Health Care for Women International* 5: 437–52
Houston, M., and P. Field. 1988. Practices and policies in the initiation of breastfeeding. *Journal of Obstetric, Gynecologic, and Neonatal Nursing* (Nov./Dec.): 418–24
Jelliffe, D. 1976. World trends in infant feeding. *American Journal of Clinical Nutrition* 29: 1227–36
Jelliffe, D., and E. Jelliffe. 1978. *Human Milk in the Modern World: Psychological, Nutritional and Economic Significance*. Toronto: Oxford University Press
– 1981. Recent trends in infant feeding. *Annual Review of Public Health* 2: 145–58
Jones, R., and E. Belsey. 1977. Breast feeding in an inner London borough: A study of cultural factors. *Social Science and Medicine* 11: 175–9

Kearney, M. 1988. Identifying psychosocial obstacles to breastfeeding success. *Journal of Obstetric, Gynecologic, and Neonatal Nursing* 17: 98–105

Keen, E. 1975. *A Primer in Phenomenological Psychology*. New York: Holt, Rinehart & Winston

Kitzinger, S. 1979. *The Experience of Breast Feeding*. New York: Penguin Books

Landsberg, M. 1982. *Women and Children First*. Markham, Ont.: Penguin Books Canada

La Rossa, R., and M. La Rossa. 1981. *Transition to Parenthood: How Infants Change Families*. Beverly Hills: Sage Publications

Lawrence, R. 1982. Practices and attitudes toward breast-feeding among medical professionals. *Pediatrics* 70: 912–20

Lee, G. S., and G. Solimano. 1981. Including mothers in the design of infant feeding research. *Studies in Family Planning* 12: 173–6

Loughlin, H., N. Clapp-Channing, S. Gehlbach, J. Pollard, and T. McCutchen. 1985. Early termination of breast-feeding: Identifying those at risk. *Pediatrics* 75: 508–13

McCaffery, M. 1984. Breastfeeding: Religious experience or hard work? *Canadian Family Physician* 30: 1441–2

Maclean, H. 1989a. Implications of a health promotion framework for research on breast feeding. *Health Promotion* 3: 355–60

– 1989b. Women's experience of breastfeeding: A much needed perspective. *Health Promotion* 3: 361–70

McNally, E., S. Hendricks, and I. Horowitz. 1985. A look at breast feeding trends in Canada (1963–1982). *Canadian Journal of Public Health* 76: 101–7

Martin, J. 1978. *Infant Feeding 1975: Attitudes and Practice in England and Wales*. London: Office of Population Censuses and Surveys, Social Survey Division, Her Majesty's Stationery Office

Marut, J., and R. Mercer. 1979. Comparison of primimaras' perceptions of vaginal and cesarean births. *Nursing Research* 28: 264

Mercer, R. 1981. The nurse and maternal tasks of early postpartum. *American Journal of Maternal Child Nursing* 6: 341–5

Miller, B., and D. Sollie. 1980. Normal stresses during the transition to parenthood. *Family Relations* 29: 459–65

Moore, I., and N. Jansa. 1987. A survey of policies and practices in support of breastfeeding mothers in the workplace. *Birth* 14: 191–5

Myres, A. 1979. A restrospective look at infant feeding practices in Canada: 1965–1978. *Journal of the Canadian Dietetic Association* 40: 200–9, 211

Oakley, A. 1979. *Becoming a Mother*. Oxford: Martin Robinson
– 1980. *Women Confined: Towards a Sociology of Childbirth*. New York: Schocken Books

Patton, M. 1980. *Qualitative Evaluation Methods*. Beverly Hills: Sage Publications

Quandt, S. 1985. Biological and behavioral predictors of exclusive breastfeeding duration. *Medical Anthropology* 7: 139–51
– 1986. Patterns of variation in breast feeding behaviours. *Social Science and Medicine* 23: 445–53

Russell, C. 1974. Transition to parenthood: Problems and gratifications. *Journal of Marriage and the Family* 36: 294–302

Sacks, S., M. Brada, and A. Hill. 1976. To breast feed or not to breast feed. *Practitioner* 216: 183–91

Sears, R., E. Maccoby, and H. Levin. 1957. *Patterns of Child Rearing*. White Plains: Harper and Row Publishers

Simopoulos, A., and G. Grave. 1984. Factors associated with the choice and duration of infant-feeding practices. Task force on infant-feeding practices. *Pediatrics* 42 (supplement): 603–14

Sjolin, S., Y. Hofvander, and C. Hillervik. 1977. Factors related to early termination of breast feeding. *Acta Paediatrica Scandinavica* 66: 505–11
– 1979. A prospective study of individual courses of breast feeding. *Acta Paediatrica Scandinavica* 68: 521–9

Sloper, K., L. McKeen, and J. Baum. 1975. Factors influencing breast feeding. *Archives of Disease in Childhood* 50: 165–70

Smith, D. 1987. *The Everyday World as Problematic: A Feminist Sociology*. Toronto: University of Toronto Press

Spradley, J. 1979. *The Ethnographic Interview*. New York: Holt, Rinehart and Winston

Sullivan, E. 1984. *A Critical Psychology: Interpretation of the Personal World*. New York: Plenum Press

Summer, G., and J. Fritsch. 1977. Postnatal parental concerns: The first six weeks of life. *Journal of Obstetric, Gynecologic and Neonatal Nursing* 6: 27–32

Tanaka, P., D. Yeung, and H. Anderson. 1987. Infant feeding practices: 1984–85 versus 1977–78. *Canadian Medical Association Journal* 136: 940–4

Taylor, S. J., and R. Bogdan. 1984. *Introduction to Qualitative Research Methods.* 2nd ed. New York: John Wiley & Sons

Tully, J., and K. Dewey. 1985. Private fears, global loss: A cross cultural study of the insufficient milk syndrome. *Medical Anthropology* 9: 225–43

Van Esterik, P., and T. Greiner. 1981. Breastfeeding and women's work: Constraints and opportunities. *Studies in Family Planning* 12: 184–97

Waletsky, L. 1977. Weaning from the breast. *World Journal of Psychosynthesis* 9: 10–14

– 1979. Breast feeding and weaning, some psychological considerations. *Primary Care* 6: 341–55

Webster's Ninth New Collegiate Dictionary. 1977. Toronto: Thomas Allen & Son

Whichelow, M. 1982. Factors associated with the duration of breast feeding in a privileged society. *Early Human Development* 7: 273–80

World Health Organization. 1981. *Contemporary Patterns of Breastfeeding: Report on the WHO Collaborative Study on Breast-feeding.* Geneva: World Health Organization

Wright, P., H. Macleod, and M. Cooper. 1983. Waking at night: The effect of early feeding experience. *Child: Care, Health and Development* 9: 309–19

Yeung, D., M. Pennell, and J. Hall. 1981. Breast feeding: Prevalence and influencing factors. *Canadian Journal of Public Health* 72: 323–30

Index

baby's temperament, 64, 116–17, 126–8, 207
body image, 39–40, 207–8
books, support, 198–9
bottle feeding: husbands' attitudes toward, 30; reasons for, 27–30; social pressure against, 25–7

decision to breast feed, 21–2

employment and breast feeding, 134–5, 138–9
engorgement, 41–2
expectations, unrealistic, 4–5, 113–16, 128–9

family, lack of support, 191–2
fatigue, 65–8, 69–71, 125
feeding routines: demand feeding, 60–2; frequency of feedings, 62–3; night feedings, 65–8; schedule feeding, 57–60; supper and evening feeding, 63–5

friends, support from, 194–5

hospital: negative experience in, 148–54; support for breast feeding, 147–8, 154–6
husbands/partners: attitudes toward breast feeding, 173–6; sharing responsibilities, 179–85

lactation consultants, 169–70
La Leche League, 195–8
leaking, 39–41
let-down, 37–8

marital relationship: changes in, 176–9, 193; sexuality, 185–90
mastitis, 42–4
milk supply: adequacy of, 127–8; arrival of, 46–7; indicators of, 47–51; insufficient, 46

night feedings, 65–8
nipple discomfort, 35–7, 125–6

persistence, 97–102
physicians: lack of support from, 51–5, 158–60, 161–3; role in early weaning, 133–4; specialist confusion, 168–9; support from, 157–8, 160–1; types of relationship with, 164–8
public breast feeding: coping with negative reactions, 86–7; social taboos, 89–91, 94; with family and friends, 83–6; with strangers, 87–91; women's changing attitudes toward, 91–3

reasons for breast feeding, 19–21
research methods, 12–14
rewards of breast feeding, 95–7, 102–7

self-esteem and breast feeding, 55–6, 117–18
socio-cultural influences, 3, 5, 22–4, 203–5
support groups, 195–8

time commitment: ambivalence about, 81–2; changes in, 205–6; ease of adjustment to, 72–82; and personal needs, 78–80, 129–30, 132–3, 136–7, 209; and relief bottle, 80; and responsibilities, 75–6
trends in breast feeding: history of, 3–4; influences on, 8–9; prevalence rates, 9–10

weaning, after four months: feelings about, 141–4; process of, 140–1; reasons for, 136–9
weaning, prior to four months: feelings after, 119–20; negative feelings about, 113–19; positive feelings about, 120–2; reasons for, 123–35
weaning, reasons for postponing, 99–101
women's experience, 4, 107–9, 210–11